GENTLE REBEL

GENTLE REBEL

THE LIFE AND WORK OF
GRANGER WESTBERG
PIONEER IN WHOLE PERSON CARE

Jane Westberg
with Jill Westberg McNamara

Church Health · Memphis, TN

ABOUT CHURCH HEALTH

Church Health seeks to reclaim the church's biblical
commitment to care for our bodies and our spirits.
Our ministries provide health care for the working
uninsured and promote healthy bodies and spirits
for all. To learn more about Church Health, visit
ChurchHealth.org. To learn more about our magazine
on health ministry, *Church Health Reader*, visit
CHReader.org.

GENTLE REBEL: THE LIFE AND WORK OF GRANGER WESTBERG
PIONEER IN WHOLE PERSON CARE
© 2015 Church Health

ISBN: 978-1-62144-049-9

Printed in the United States of America

Church Health is proud to publish this resource using
recycled materials.

Design by Lizy Heard

Contents

Foreword

I **first briefly met Granger Westberg** as the father of a college classmate, who happens to be the author of this biography. I got to know him much better two years later when I went to see him in his capacity as chaplain at the University of Chicago where he had joint appointments on the medical and divinity school faculties.

At that point I was a student in the Divinity School, and my childhood faith was being strongly tested by the intense and probing intellectual atmosphere at the Divinity School. I was upset, both physically and emotionally, and I sought Granger's counsel. His gentle physical presence, kind smile, and soothing voice were immediately therapeutic. His insights about the nature of my struggle—and his reassurance about the normalcy of what I was experiencing—were more effective than any pill or platitude could possibly have been. Our dialogue that year became the basis for a lifelong friendship.

I assume that hundreds, if not thousands, of individuals had similar encounters with Granger during his lifetime of teaching and healing. And, after being reminded in this wonderful biography of his many leadership roles in transforming health care both in and out of the hospital, I am sure he indirectly touched the lives of many more.

Individuals who met or worked with Granger were shaped by his vision for a transformed experience of health care. Countless clergy, nurses, and physicians, even many who never met Granger, felt the impact of his life's work in the quality of their education and in the expectations shaping their ongoing work. And countless organizations have and are being influenced by his conviction that the church could do a better job of offering ministries that heal lives, medically as well as spiritually.

Peace to his memory.
G. Timothy Johnson, MD

Introduction

For as long as he or anyone in our family could remember, my father, Granger Westberg, wanted to be a minister. As a four-year-old, he would make a pulpit out of a large chair by turning it around so the back of it faced his audience. Then he would stand on the chair and begin preaching, waving his hands as he had seen ministers do.

Dad did become a minister, but his career was far from conventional. He loved the church, but he had a vision of it being even more relevant, compassionate, and healing. In the 1940s, he began thinking about the body, mind, and spirit, along with ways that ministers and churches could partner with doctors and nurses in providing whole person care. Wholistic Health Centers and parish nurses (later, faith community nurses) were two models he pioneered for providing this kind of care. Dad also had ideas about the ways that seminaries and schools in the health professions could better prepare people to provide whole person care.

As an irrepressibly optimistic innovator, he sometimes was dismayed when people were not yet ready to share his excitement about new ideas and ventures. Resistance, however, seldom stopped him. He wasn't confrontational, but he persisted.

Why, I wondered, did my father become a maverick minister? What led him into whole person care seven decades ago when that concept was rarely thought of, let alone discussed? What gave him the courage to challenge assumptions and traditions? In a day when doctors were authority figures on pedestals, what led him to think doctors would come to accept clergy as members of health teams? What contributed to his incredible capacity to generate new ideas and envision a better future? What enabled him to be optimistic and continue trying to "sell" his ideas, even in the face of substantial obstacles?

In an attempt to answer these and other questions, in what turned out to be the last two years of his life, I asked my father to retell some of the stories of his childhood that he had told my brother and me when he tucked us in at night. I also asked him to tell me stories from his later life and career. I audiotaped some of these accounts, and together we read and discussed his published articles, unpublished manuscripts, and even his handwritten notes and old photos. I also talked at length with some of Dad's colleagues, and others who knew him and his work. In addition, I did library research. As I began drafting this manuscript, Dad carefully reviewed what I wrote.

After Dad's death, I left the manuscript alone for many years, but thanks to my siblings, particularly Jill, we worked on Dad's story from time to time. Then, with the support of the Church Health Center, we finally finished the project.

Many of the stories in this book are in Dad's voice. I quote from his writings and from the audiotapes of him retelling his stories. (In fact, throughout the book, quotations that are not referenced are from the audio recordings.) Even though I did careful research for this book, I cannot claim to have written a full, definitive, objective biography. I tell his life as I witnessed it and heard about it from him and others. My hope is to share his remarkable life and achievements. I want people to be inspired so that they might also question assumptions, envision creative alternatives, and work at healing the wounds in this world, making it a more compassionate, love-giving, health-promoting place. And to do it gently and with kindness to others, as Dad did.

Chapter 1

Only the Beginning

In the autumn of 1993, my 80-year-old father and I arrived a little late at the hotel where the seventh annual Westberg Symposium was getting started. Dad always liked to arrive early at events, but he was moving slowly that day because of the challenges of Parkinson's disease. Once in the hotel we locked arms so he could walk as fast as possible. When we quietly opened a side door, hoping to slip unnoticed into the back of the large room, the speaker was already addressing the 400 or so parish nurses and other participants. As the speaker saw Dad enter, she stopped mid-sentence and almost reverentially announced his presence. There was an audible gasp as everyone stood up and strained to see him. Then they began applauding while people near the door offered us their seats. When Dad and I looked at each other, we both had tears in our eyes.

Throughout the conference, whenever there was a break between sessions and crowds were milling about, I had no trouble locating Dad. He was always in the middle of an admiring group of nurses. No wonder he always came home from the symposia walking on air.

At one event, all of us participants were seated around small tables and given a sheet of paper with a large circle. Our task was to draw with crayons our vision of the future. When we showed our drawings to each other, most people had stayed within the circle, but Dad had drawn circles that spiraled out of the original circle and reached to all the edges of the paper. He had written, "Only the beginning."

Granger Westberg was born July 11, 1913 to Alma Ahlstrom and John Westberg in their modest home in a Swedish and Norwegian community on the southwest side of Chicago. His father, his two sisters (13-year-old Viola and seven-year-old Eulalia, called "Lael"), and his five-year-old brother, Orville, had waited restlessly all day. In the next few days Granger was also welcomed by other members of his close-knit family, including aunts, uncles, and cousins from both his mother's and father's sides of the family.

Of all of the people shaping young Granger's life, his mother, Alma, was the most powerful. In fact, she probably remained one of the strongest influences on him throughout his life. In his 80s Granger said that hardly a day had gone by that he hadn't thought of her.

Alma was a great student of the Bible and read her devotional literature every night. As a pietistic Lutheran she felt it was her duty to bring her children up in "the faith" and ensure they would all be reunited in heaven. Toward this end, she made sure that the family always said grace before each meal and had devotions at the family altar each night. She also cautioned them not to break the Ten Commandments and forbid them to engage in such "worldly" activities as dancing, playing cards, and attending movies. Alma was very active in the church and took the children to Sunday services and other events.

There were a lot of "thou-shalt-nots" in Alma's vocabulary, so it was easy for energetic, inquisitive Granger to get into trouble. Almost always, naughty behavior resulted in a verbal spanking. Sometimes, while Granger was still smaller than his five-foot, one-inch mother, she gave him physical spankings as well—or at least she tried to. When she would reach out to spank him, he would start running around the house. More than once as Alma was chasing him around the dining room table, he made her laugh with his antics. Early on, he realized that he could deflect his mother's negativity and anger with charm and humor. This strategy served him well in later years, both with his mother and with other people in positions of authority.

Alma was a bright, strong-minded woman, but she also presented herself as delicate and in need of care. Granger, like others, could be solicitous when Alma complained of her nervous stomach and other problems, but he grew to be embarrassed by her preoccupation with her health. He was upset when family plans had to be adjusted to Alma's illnesses. Alma's attitudes and behaviors were likely factors in Granger's interest in learning more about the mind-body relationship. Later in life, Granger hypothesized that his mother, who lived to be 96, would probably have had a different focus in her life had she been able to go to high school rather than work to help support her immigrant family.

Granger's father John, a Swedish immigrant, helped shape Granger's life in quiet ways. John was tender and loving, often calling Granger, *min lilla vän* (Swedish for "my little friend"). John was a man of few words and a little hard to get to know, but as Granger grew older it became clear to him that his father was well loved, not only by his immediate family but also by the extended family. In fact, it was said that in times of death of loved ones, family members would call John before calling the undertaker. John was the family's anchor.

As a young boy, Granger enjoyed going to work with his father at the large sash and door company where John was the manager and often functioned also as president. Granger was sure the workers allowed him to do some fun little jobs and treated him with respect because they thought so highly of his father. Later Granger realized that his father was widely acknowledged in the business world for his honesty and fairness with customers, workers, and other business people.

John was an active church member, but unlike Alma, he was more open to other ways of thinking. He was also part of the Swedish-American secular life in Chicago. Granger enjoyed hearing his father talk about events at the South Side Swedish Club and the singing clubs to which he belonged.

Because of his impeccable reputation as a businessman, Granger's father served on the board of directors of Augustana Hospital, an institution of the Augustana Lutheran Synod on the north side of Chicago. At the supper table Granger heard many conversations about the hospital. Early on he learned from his father that caring for the sick was a central responsibility of the church.

As the baby of the family, Granger got lots of attention, particularly from Viola. Granger: "My mother was ill a lot, so Viola was like a second mother to me. She was such a loving person. You couldn't help but love her. She never got angry. She was comforting and sweet. But she'd say what she thought when the occasion called for it."

Lael also looked after her little brother and over the years became increasingly important in his life. Granger looked up to his big brother, Orville, who was handsome and musical.

Viola, Lael, and Orville had many friends and were involved in activities out of the house. Granger: "I was eager to be included, so as Viola and Lael were leaving the house for a date or Orville was leaving to do something fun, I frequently begged, 'Can I go too?' In fact, I asked that question so often that I was called 'Little Can I Go Too Westberg.'"

The sound of music in the Westberg house was almost continuous. Music was an important form of communication, pleasure, and recognition. By the time Granger was ready to study an instrument, Viola was teaching 40 piano students at the family house. Granger: "Viola tried to teach me to play the piano, but she was my sister, not my parent, so I didn't feel that I needed to do what she told me. Also, the piano was almost never available because my sisters and Viola's students were using it all the time."

Granger was more comfortable singing: "Our family sang a lot at home. Sometimes we gathered around the piano as Viola accompanied us. On family car trips or while doing dishes we sang a cappella, harmonizing to favorite songs."

Born to the Church

When Granger was an infant, Alma dressed blond-haired, hazel-eyed Granger in the family's long white lace baptismal gown. The proud family took him to nearby Bethel Lutheran Church, which his parents, maternal grandparents, and others helped found before the turn of the century. There Pastor Andrew Fors baptized Granger into the church community.

Bethel was the Westberg family's second home. "We would never think of not going to church," Granger said. As a small boy he attended Sunday school, where he listened to Bible stories, sang songs such as "Jesus Loves Me," and memorized Bible verses. Granger also went to Sunday services where the minister's "hell, fire, and brimstone" preaching sometimes frightened him. Later in life he wrote:[1]

> I grew up in Chicago and with my family attended a large church that had the highest ceilings a little boy ever thought a church could have. Written in large Gothic type, high above a main window in the nave, were the words, "The fear of the Lord is the beginning of wisdom." Frequently, the solemn-faced pastor, with a dramatic gesture and booming voice, would shout out these words, particularly the word *fear*, so as to curdle my blood. It was the fear and the power of this God that made me shake in my shoes. It didn't help either that in the stained glass window immediately below those words was the huge symbol of the all-seeing eye of God. And that eye was always looking down on me to catch me if I broke any of his laws.
>
> The pastor compounded the problem by shouting those words from a pulpit that appeared to me to be two stories high. I envisioned the pastor as having just talked to God, like Moses on the mount.

Fortunately, family members surrounded Granger during church services. His parents sang in the choir, along with Alma's sister

Marie, Marie's husband, and other relatives. Granger's Uncle Will (one of his father's brothers) was the director of the large choir. Will also played the organ until Viola took over that position.

Granger's family was involved in church activities throughout the week. Alma and John went to choir practice. Alma was active in the missionary society and other organizations. For 26 years, Granger's father was secretary of the church. Often he was a delegate to meetings of the Illinois Conference of Augustana Lutheran churches and to the national meetings of the Lutheran Augustana Synod, which had been founded by Swedish immigrants, particularly ministers of the Church of Sweden.[2] Granger's siblings attended youth activities. Sometimes Alma took Granger with her to church prayer services.

On Christmas Eve, Alma's side of the family came together to eat their favorite traditional Swedish holiday food, read the ancient scriptures, sing Christmas carols, and open the brightly decorated gifts under the Christmas tree. They also went to church for the pageant and a service. Granger: "For several years I was a shepherd in the Christmas Eve pageant at church. I wore a bathrobe. I didn't have much to say, only, 'Glory to God in the highest.'"

At four o'clock Christmas morning, the family was back in church for the julotta (sunrise) service. Then the large Westberg clan gathered for the smorgasbord breakfast feast at the Westberg house featuring treats from "the old country."

Whenever the Westbergs gathered, whether at Christmas or another time, they made music in what essentially was an extended family choir. The 20–30 family members sang, accompanied on the piano by Viola and directed by Granger's Uncle Will. Sometimes another uncle played the violin.

At age 13, Granger, became a member of the confirmation class, which was designed to prepare children who had reached "the age of reason" for a public examination that enabled them to be full adult members of the church. During confirmation class, the children memorized Martin Luther's *Small Catechism*, which included the

Apostles' Creed and Luther's understandings of the meanings of these documents. There was no room for questioning.

When Granger began confirmation classes, Pastor Fors broke with the tradition of having the minister as the sole teacher. Instead, he divided the class into boys and girls. He instructed the boys, while Granger's 20-year-old-sister, Lael, did most of the teaching of the girls. Unfortunately, from Granger's point of view, Pastor Fors retained the tradition of mindless memorization. Granger wished that he could have been in Lael's class because she welcomed students' questions: "If girls in those days had been allowed to go into the ministry, I think Lael would have become a minister. She always had a keen interest in theology. The girls in her class were so enthusiastic and loved her so much that most of them continued to meet monthly for 40 years. She opened their minds like she opened my mind."

Granger had an active, questioning mind. Lael appreciated his questions, and the two of them frequently talked far into the night. In fact, both when he was younger and later in his career, Granger regarded Lael as his mentor.

As in other Augustana Synod churches, on the day of his confirmation, Granger and the other students were quizzed in front of the congregation during a Sunday service. In essence, they recited what they had memorized. Then they knelt at the altar railing to receive their first communion. In his 80s Granger still had a vivid memory of his first communion: "I remember being bothered by the way some of the other boys in the class giggled during communion. I felt they were desecrating the sacrament. When it was my turn to sip from the cup of wine, I was in for a shock. No one told me how strong wine was, and I spilled some when I drank it. That made me very embarrassed. I was very moved and impressed by the service, so much so that when I became a pastor, my hands would shake with emotion as I gave communion to the first table of people."

Shortly after Granger was confirmed, Pastor C. Emil Bergquist became Bethel's new pastor. Late in life Granger remembered:[3]

He was wonderful, bright, warm, and loved by the people. I was very lucky because right away he took me under his wing. The first Sunday he preached about Solomon. After the service, I went up to him and asked, 'How could Solomon be a wonderful man if he had 1,000 wives?' 'Good question,' he said, 'Let's talk about it. Why don't we meet in my study?' I couldn't believe that my pastor was inviting me to talk with him. But he was. When we got together we talked about everything. He loved questions and discussions.

This was only the beginning of many meaningful conversations. Pastor Bergquist was warm and listened attentively I felt that he cared for me and for other members of the congregation with whom he also spent time. He really wanted to get to know us. Because I wanted to be a minister, he later translated a book called *Soul Care* for me from Swedish. Each time we met, we'd discuss a new chapter.

Pastor Bergquist arrived in Granger's life at an important time. Granger loved the church, but there were some things that bothered him greatly. Granger: "I felt hemmed in when I was with people who weren't open to other ways of thinking. I wanted to move out into the real world. Bergquist helped me realize that I could be myself. He was very independent. He allowed for the church to be open to diversity."

Restless for the Future

Granger remained loyal to his church. After his confirmation, he joined the Luther League—a nationwide program for young people that had a branch in most Augustana churches. He was also an active member of the church's Boy Scouts troop. But Granger wanted more, and he wanted alternatives to some of what bothered him in his own church. Rather than just complaining, he actively sought out other ways of doing things.

Granger felt comfortable in the YMCA (Young Men's Christian

Association): "There was a quality of interest shown to me personally by people in the Y which was shown by no one else in my teens except my pastor. The teachers were intelligent and made learning fun. Many of them were good athletes who could handle themselves in just about every sport. That was appealing to a teen-aged boy."

Another source of nourishment was the music at a local Episcopal Church. Granger:

> I was told that St. Bartholomew Episcopal Church had a wonderful choir with about 20 boys and 20 men. I went there and found that it was just like the choirs of the great cathedrals, so I joined the choir. The first Sunday that we sang the Kyrie was the closest I've ever come to the expression "being saved." Later, when evangelicals asked me if I had been saved. I would say, "Yes." When I told them that it was at the Episcopal Church, they weren't very happy. They would pray for me that I might see the light.
>
> My mother couldn't figure out what I was doing. I finally got my dad to come to St. Bartholomew's. He liked it. He said that it reminded him of the cathedral in his parish in Sweden.
>
> The rector of the Episcopal church used to kid me a bit. He'd say, "Are you going to be a Lutheran pastor or an Episcopal priest? You think real hard about it, because we would like to have you."
>
> Pastor Bergquist was not bothered by my going to another church. I was intrigued with the Episcopal church, but the Lutheran church was my spiritual home where I cherished being with family.

The Great Depression Hits Home

When Granger entered high school, his father's business was doing well. In 1927, however, the real estate market had lost its buoyancy. Then on Black Thursday, October 24, 1929, the stock market crashed.

Panic struck the city. Granger: "Thousands of people were out of work. Twice each week, our pastor and many volunteers provided meals for people who were having difficulties. My father helped with this, and he also helped set up a little insurance program called Bethel Sick Benefit Society."

In the spring of 1931, John Westberg's business was in serious trouble. The company was in the business of helping to construct businesses and homes, but, as the Depression deepened, new construction declined severely. More and more businesses closed. Hundreds of Chicagoans were evicted from their homes each week. Those who didn't have any place to stay had to construct makeshift homes out of corrugated tin or whatever they could find.

Although he hated to interrupt Orville's senior year at the University of Idaho, John asked his son if he'd come home and help with the business. Orville, who planned to take over the business, returned home and worked frantically with his father to keep the business alive. Granger wanted to help, but he didn't have the needed skills. The family urged him to stay in school.

When Granger graduated from Calumet High School, he wanted to go to Augustana College in Rock Island, Illinois. With the family's financial problems, however, Granger had to abandon his dream. Granger: "When my counselor at Calumet High School learned that I was interested in the ministry and needed to attend a reasonably-priced college, she recommended George Williams College. The college was a 45-minute streetcar ride from home, just north of the University of Chicago, so I could save money by living at home."

Jobs were scarce the summer before Granger started college, but he was able to work as a lifeguard at the Augustana Synod church camp at Long Lake. Every summer since he was 12, Granger had been a camper. He particularly had enjoyed swimming and pillow fights. Now he supervised swimmers and refereed pillow fights.

During that summer, following Lael's suggestion, Granger also took courses in shorthand and typing. As a young man beginning college in the early years of the Depression, he might not have realized how much these skills would serve him for the rest of his life when he typed his sermons, his articles for publication and an endless flow of proposals for innovative projects.

Chapter 2

Fast Talking

The Depression and its growing impact on the family took a little of the joy out of Granger's freshman year at George Williams College, an all-men's school established to educate men for work in the YMCA. But optimistic Granger enjoyed the people and his classes and felt he got a lot out of his first college year. Decades later when Granger gave talks on whole person care, he acknowledged his indebtedness to the YMCA for their triangular symbol with the words "body, mind and spirit" that helped him develop his understanding of wholism. He used this triangle in his chalk talks, a common method at the time for giving talks with visual support through drawings made by the speaker while the audience watched. Granger also reflected that the school's focus on good health habits probably contributed to his later interest in preventive medicine.

During his freshman year, Granger also enjoyed spending time with Lael and Orville, who were living at home with him and his parents. Lael was working for Professor Fred Eastman at Chicago Theological Seminary. She and Granger talked about what Lael was learning in the liberal seminary community. Before the school year was out, Lael began speaking with Granger about a bright young theological student who quickly became the love of her life. Daniel Day Williams was also to become an important person in Granger's life, as well as in the lives of many theology students and others all over the world.

Conversations with Orville focused on trying to help their father save the company. Granger:

> By cutting his own salary and taking other economic measures, my father had managed to keep his business afloat. However, members of one of the carpenters unions in Chicago wanted Dad to raise his employees' salaries. Dad wanted to, but because of the Depression he couldn't afford to do that without going bankrupt. Dad was willing to give his employees a raise on paper and pay them later when the company was in better financial shape.
>
> All of my father's employees had agreed with this plan, except a new employee whom we later learned was a "union steward" working undercover in the company and trying to stir up trouble among the employees. One day, just in time, an employee found an incendiary device that had been planted in the engine room. Had he not spotted it, it would have blown up some of the machinery and maybe hurt or killed someone.
>
> Later four thugs, who were hired by the union, "visited" my father, telling him he had to raise his employees' salaries "or else." My father again told them what the situation was. They said, "Well, that's your tough luck." With that, the union called a strike that closed the company.

Reflecting in his 80s on this event, Granger said, "This experience caused me to have some negative feelings about unions. But I have been in favor of them for the most part. Many heads of businesses take too much for themselves and leave little for their employees. My father, though, took very little for himself. He had about 50 employees, some of whom were family members. He was paying top rates to all of them, but the unions wanted him to pay them even more. Going out of business meant the end of all of their livelihoods. My father was a very honest and kind man. I never heard him yell. He didn't belong in that business world."

Although Granger's father was of retirement age when his company went under, he got a job as a consultant to a lumber company located outside of Chicago. Between that work and contributions from Orville and Lael, the family was able to keep their house and have food on the table.

Augustana-Bound

Although Granger felt positively about his education at George Williams, his goal had been to go to Augustana College. At the end of his freshmen year, with his family's approval, Granger decided to transfer to Augustana College. To help pay for his expenses, that summer Granger again worked as a lifeguard, this time at a camp for inner city Chicago children operated by the social ministry of the Illinois Conference of the Augustana Lutheran Synod. The camp was located on beautiful Lake Geneva in Wisconsin. Granger earned only five dollars a week, plus board and room, but he felt lucky to have a job.

Granger was interested in "what makes people tick," so he majored in psychology at Augustana. Viola's husband's parents helped Granger with his college expenses by letting him stay in a small bedroom in their house in nearby Moline, Illinois. To pay for his tuition, books, food, and other needs, Granger juggled several jobs with a full load of classes. One of his jobs was on the college campus, serving for about two hours each day as a janitor: "I was responsible for cleaning the women's dorm. I got kidded a lot about that job," he said. Granger also applied for work at Mosenfelder's Men's Store in Rock Island, where his stylish brother, Orville, had worked during his two years at Augustana. Granger: "I told them that Orville was my brother. They had liked him a lot, so they gave me a job. I worked there from 9:00 a.m. until 9:00 p.m. every Saturday. At noon I would have a $.25 vegetarian meal at the 5 and 10-cent store across the street. Unfortunately, the college football games were on Saturdays, so I missed them."

Two afternoons a week Granger worked as a lifeguard and swimming teacher at a nearby YMCA. He also rehearsed and directed the children's choir at an Episcopal church in Rock Island. Granger: "After the service, the rector brought the offering plates back to the sacristy. He'd pick up $.75 and give that to me. That was my pay. He also suggested that I buy a pair of clear glasses to wear to give me an older look. I got a pair at a 5 and 10-cent store and wore them every Sunday."

In his first year at Augustana, Granger successfully auditioned as a baritone for the Augustana Choir, directed by Henry Veld. Granger: "I had to choose between being in the choir or going out for the basketball team. I'm glad I chose being in the choir because it was at the peak of its popularity, singing in famous places such as Carnegie Hall in New York and Orchestra Hall in Chicago. We rehearsed several days a week. I was in the choir all three years I was at Augustana College and the first year I was in seminary."

In the era of college pranks, Granger remembered: "We had fun. Before one of the performances, some of the men in the choir deliberately ate garlic. Since they stood behind the women during the performance, the women could smell the garlic but they couldn't laugh or do anything about it while we were singing in front of an audience."

Granger was raised with a sense of mission. Feeling that the people of Rock Island and the region should have access to fine music, Granger, with Dr. Veld's approval, talked the local radio station manager into broadcasting the choir's performances. Granger hosted these broadcasts.

Meeting His Match

At the beginning of his junior year, after being at Augustana for only one year, Granger was elected class president. One October day, during his junior year, he recalled: "I was studying in the library next to my friend Stewart Weinstein ('Abie') when I saw a beautiful brunette across the room. I asked Abie if he knew her. He said, 'Sure that's Helen Johnson. I went to Davenport High School with her.' When I told Abie that I'd like to ask her out, he told me to forget it because Helen was dating Don Smiley, captain of Augie's football team."

Granger decided to try anyway and managed to snag a date with Helen. Helen, who lived in Davenport, Iowa, recalled: "We couldn't leave my house because the weather was so terrible. Heaven and earth froze together the night of our first date. But my mother didn't invite Granger to stay overnight. He didn't have a car, so he had to return the same way he came, by three slow-moving streetcars, one of which crossed the Mississippi River back to Rock Island."

That night Helen wrote in her diary: "Had a date with a fellow from Chicago. He's president of our class. Very nice, but cocky."

Granger recalled, "Helen felt sorry for me for how things went that first night, so she went out of her way to be nice to me." Helen's mother invited Granger back for many bountiful meals at the Johnson household. Included at the table were Helen's older sister Elizabeth, her younger sister Jean, and Helen's father, "O. E.," a popular physical education teacher at Helen's alma mater, Davenport High School.

With his very limited income, Granger survived on oatmeal and other inexpensive foods, so he welcomed opportunities to feast at the Johnsons' on pot roast, vegetables, mashed potatoes, and custard pies. And he liked the Johnsons. Granger: "I enjoyed getting to know Helen's family. Her mother was warm and friendly. I particularly remember her hearty laugh and her jolly voice when she talked on the telephone."

After a few dates Granger, eager to impress Helen, offered to teach her to swim in the college pool. As a lifeguard he had a key. They went to the pool after hours—alone. At the pool Granger showed Helen how to blow bubbles, breathe correctly, and kick while holding onto the side of the pool. After giving her these instructions, Granger told Helen to stay in the shallow water and practice while he swam in the deep end. He hoisted himself out of the pool. As he walked toward the deep end of the pool, Helen sprinted in a perfect crawl stroke to the deep end. Granger stopped in his tracks as Helen passed him.

Granger had neglected to ask Helen if she could swim. In fact, Helen was an excellent swimmer and probably could have taught Granger a thing or two. For many summers, she had spent a good deal of time at the Davenport Natatorium where her father was the summer manager. She had recently won the Tri City free-style event.

As Helen and Granger's relationship progressed, Helen's parents did not say much about Granger. According to Helen, "That meant that they approved of him." Later when Helen and Granger's relationship became more serious, Helen's mother, Marie, did caution Helen about marrying a Lutheran. The Johnsons were active in and proud of their church—First Presbyterian Church of Davenport.

During the summer after his junior year Granger, who continually needed to scramble for money, demonstrated Health-o-Meter Bathroom Scales at a booth at Chicago's second World's Fair. He became an effective hawker, calling and singing out his invitation for people to try the scales that came in black, white, blue, green, orchid, pink, and yellow. His sales pitch was so much fun that for decades family and friends asked him to repeat it.

Granger needed his fast talking skills in another arena. In his and other Lutheran families, a marriage even between a Swedish Lutheran and a Danish Lutheran was considered a "mixed marriage," so he was concerned how his mother would react to his dating Helen, a non-Scandinavian Presbyterian. Granger: "When I told my parents about Helen and her family, they were impressed. They were even more impressed when they learned that her father was a long-time Sunday school teacher. When they asked if Helen was Swedish, I sidestepped the question a bit and said, 'Her last name is Johnson.' (Johnson could be a Swedish name.)"

It probably also helped that Lael was dating Dan Williams, a Congregational seminarian whom the family loved dearly. Six decades later, Granger reflected: "Over the years it became clear that my mother was not strongly denominational. She just wanted to be sure that the church 'preached Christ.'"

The summer that Granger worked at the World's Fair, he had an opportunity to introduce his parents and Helen to one another. Helen recalled, "Granger's family made me feel very welcome. Later his mother even took my side when Granger and I had disagreements."

Continued Stirrings against Conformity

During college, Granger had growing doubts about whether to enter the ministry. Later, reflecting on his college days in an article titled "Are Ministers in a Rut?," Granger wrote:[1]

> In my more cynical moments as a college student, I felt that ministers were pretty much in a rut ... I felt certain that there was little freedom of thought in theological education, for most ministers seemed to have come out of the same mold.
>
> While I know now that I was hypercritical in my attitude—and also full of youthful arrogance ... if, while in college, I had not felt some stirrings against this conformity, I would not have entered the seminary.

Fortunately, while at church camp, Granger had heard a talk given by Claus A. Wendell, an Augustana Lutheran who was pastor to the students at the University of Minnesota. Granger said that Wendell was considered a radical in his day because, "he refused to be fenced in or to be told that there was only one way to come at answers to questions."

Dr. Wendell felt that many things needed to be changed, and he said so, but always with tangible suggestions of how the change could be brought about. As a pastor of students on a college campus, Dr. Wendell was ecumenical. That appealed to me because I liked to get the perspectives of other denominations.

Dr. Wendell demonstrated that a Christian pastor can be a severe critic of the Church and yet do it in a most constructive manner. One of the reasons that I and several other college students went into the ministry was that Dr. Wendell and several leaders within the Augustana Church assured us that as clergy we could still be ourselves and be open to new ways of thinking.[2]

On June 4, 1935 Helen and Granger graduated from Augustana College. Two days later, Granger's brother, Orville, married Ruth Johnson, a young woman of Swedish descent whom he met while attending the University of Idaho, where he went to school after trying to help his father with the business. Seven days after Orville and Ruth's wedding, Lael married Daniel Day Williams in New York City, where Dan was working on his doctorate in philosophy at Columbia University. Granger and the other family members could not afford to travel to the wedding. Granger and a friend, however, did pay Lael and Dan a surprise visit when they took a detour during their summer jobs driving cars between states and turned up where the newlyweds were spending their honeymoon.

Some of Granger and Helen's college friends also were getting married that summer, but Granger and Helen could not afford to be married. Granger was facing four years of study at Augustana Seminary, and the seminary faculty strongly recommended that seminarians remain single so they could focus their energy on their studies. In fact, to discourage the marriage of seminarians, the seminary only gave single men free tuition. (There were no female seminarians and it would be a long time before women were accepted into the seminary and ordained.)[3]

Also, if Granger and Helen had married straight out of college, it would have been very difficult for Helen to get a job. In general, women had far fewer job opportunities than men because employers and the general public thought women should not take jobs away from men. Married women had even more trouble getting jobs than single women because it was widely believed that married men should support their wives.

As it turned out, even as a single woman with a degree in history and the intention to become a teacher, Helen couldn't get a job as a teacher. The summer after graduation, she had to settle for a job at a bakery where she earned only $2.00 for each long day's work.

Chapter 3

The Larger Vision

In the fall of 1935, Granger entered Augustana Theological Seminary. Fortunately the seminary was being transformed from a "preacher factory" to a more academic institution. From 1900 to 1930, with one exception, no professor at Augustana Seminary possessed a bona fide PhD degree. None of them had done significant research. The faculty, elected by the Augustana Synod, were chiefly pastors who had distinguished themselves as popular preachers or competent administrators of church affairs but had no scholarly achievements.

Following protests from seminary students, four professors were relieved of their responsibilities at the end of the 1930–1931 school year. Four new professors (Conrad E. Bergendoff, Alvin D. Mattson, Erik H. Wahlstrom, and Carl A. Anderson), with academic credentials, were hired.[1]

Granger saw more ways that theological education could be improved. Later in life he recalled:

> I never learned Hebrew and Greek well enough to read intelligently. When we studied the Scriptures in those languages, we'd spend more time translating than studying the Scriptures. I would have preferred sticking with good English translations. In fact, years later when I was a member of the board of Augustana College and Seminary, the first thing I proposed was teaching

Greek and Hebrew during the summer in the three months before seminary began. Parts of that proposal were accepted.

There was a major effort to make the academics sound. Teaching was mostly by straight lectures, but since there were only 16 of us in my class, there were opportunities for discussions among students and faculty. Most of us lived in the same dorm, so our bull sessions continued after class. Night after night we were stimulated by our requirement that if you took a stand, you had to defend it.

Every school day, seminarians were expected to attend chapel services. Granger learned that no musician was available to play the piano or organ for the services. He recalled, "I agreed to play the piano as long as none of the hymns had more than two sharps. I could play pieces in keys with one or two sharps, but more sharps than that was too difficult for me."[2] With his continuing sense of the power of worship and with many ideas about ways to improve worship services, 22-year-old Granger, wrote a series of articles on "The Art of Worship" for *The Lutheran Companion*, the national journal of the Augustana Lutheran Synod.[3] He was very young to be making these kinds of suggestions to his elders, but that obviously didn't stop him.

During seminary, Granger and some other seminarians were eager to hear fresh perspectives and have their thinking challenged. Granger had been so impressed with Claus A. Wendell when he heard him speak years earlier that he talked the group into inviting Wendell to speak at the seminary. Since conservatives had branded Wendell as a heretic, Granger was considered daring to invite him to speak. Many years after seminary, Granger wrote:[4]

We all looked forward to hearing this pastor because we knew he had been forced off the faculty of a Lutheran Bible Institute after writing a small book entitled, *The Larger Vision*,[5] which was an attempt to show that the world had probably been created over a longer period that just six days.

Wendall had long been a pastor to Lutheran students at the University of Minnesota where it was known that he spent most of his time sitting around with publicans and sinners and scientists. He not only believed that the world was round but he believed that Charles Darwin had opened a few windows that needed opening.

Having heard so many rumors about Wendell, the seminary students expected a fiery man filled with rebellion. Instead, they saw a kindly, gray-haired, soft-spoken man who refused the use of the lectern and just sat down and swapped stories with us. I guess he actually gave his speech but he did it in little bits in response to what the fellows wanted to know.

Speaking further of Wendell, Granger wrote: "He did not make us feel that we had to compartmentalize religion and the ideas of this world. He was not defensive at any point. He seemed to have no fear of being completely open about stating what he believed. It was easy to understand how he got along so well with people outside the church. It was depressing to us to realize that such an honest man could not be accepted, just as he was, inside the church."[6]

It's difficult to know how many people shared Granger's reaction. Clearly, Granger was hungry for change and learned both from the content and the process of Wendell's presentation.

Back home in Chicago, Pastor Bergquist continued to support Granger: "When I went home for Christmas or Easter, he would ask me to assist with the liturgy. Sometimes he'd invite me to preach. I had to do all of this in front of my relatives. They were okay though. After a while, they even started saying, 'You're getting to be a pretty good preacher.'

"Much later while I was at the University of Chicago Hospital, I became Bergquist's chaplain when he was ill. His physician hadn't picked up on his problem early enough, so by the time he got to the university hospital, it was too late. He was a relatively young man when he died. I still miss him."

A Year Apart

In 1934, Augustana Seminary became one of the first seminaries in the United States to extend its program to four years. They did this by adding one year of parish service that students were required to take after two years of residence at the seminary. Following this so-called "internship," students returned to the seminary for their senior year. Later, Granger was to be a strong advocate for including clinical experiences in theological education. However, this change in the curriculum apparently occurred not because the faculty decided it was important for seminarians to have real world experiences, but because the Great Depression had so reduced congregational incomes that many churches could not afford a pastor.[7]

In the autumn of 1938, Granger was assigned to Greendale Lutheran Church in Worcester, Massachusetts, for his one-year internship. Granger's supervising pastor, Martin Luther Cornell, was the president (a position comparable to bishop) of the New England Conference of the Augustana Lutheran Church. Granger: "In September, Martin Cornell had a call to a church in St. Paul, Minnesota. In late October he left, so I had the church all by myself. I enjoyed the work, and being on my own gave me a sense of the responsibilities facing pastors. In retrospect, though, I think I would have learned even more if I had some good feedback and supervision."

While Granger was in Worcester, Helen was dealing with a tough assignment. She had finally secured a job teaching fourth, fifth, and sixth grade social studies at the local Iowa Soldiers and Sailors State Orphanage. Her monthly salary was $60.00. Helen: "Only about two dozen of the 800 children were orphans. Many of the others qualified for reform school. They had been taken from their homes because of serious problems. I taught in different classrooms. The kids referred to Florida Flemming, the teacher I followed from room to room, as 'Florida Flip Flop.' Florida left the classroom in such bedlam that sometimes when I walked in the kids were jumping from desktop to desktop. One day I found a butcher knife in a girl's desk. This was the same type of knife the girl had used to kill her mother."

Helen was very bothered by how the children were disciplined: "The teachers would rap the children's knuckles or spank them." Once a week, Helen had "cottage duty." She read to the 37 11-year-old boys, who were in her charge, and then put them to bed. "It wasn't an easy job, and there were no opportunities for giving individual attention to the boys," Helen recalled.

Granger and Helen knew that they needed Helen's income. Granger wished they were together so he could give her more support.

Fortunately Granger was able to look forward to Helen's visit to Worcester at Christmas. It was to be her first trip to New England, and she and Granger had agreed that they would become engaged during the visit.

In Worcester Helen attended the Christmas service and heard Granger give a short greeting in Swedish before conducting the rest of the service in English. Shortly after Christmas, Granger and Helen drove into Boston, which still gleamed with holiday lights. Their most important mission was selecting an engagement ring. They also traveled to New York City where they fulfilled a long-held dream to attend a symphony at Carnegie Hall and to visit Radio City Music Hall, home of the Rockettes (a showgirl-style dancing ensemble).

After Christmas, Helen went back home with an engagement ring on her finger, and the new pastor arrived at Greendale Lutheran Church in Worcester. Apparently the new pastor wasn't prepared to deal with an intern, so Granger needed to move on. More than 350 people attended a farewell reception for him and presented him with money and a traveling bag.

Granger: "The seminary didn't know what to do with me, so they sent me down to the vice president of the New England Conference [of the Augustana Synod], who at that time was pastor of a huge church in Hartford, Connecticut. I stayed with him for two weeks, helping him write the presidential annual report to the synod. Then I was asked to serve a new little congregation of about 40 members in New Bedford, Massachusetts. It quickly became clear that New Bedford couldn't support two Lutheran churches, so we began merging the churches and building the attendance. I really got a thrill out of it, but after I left, I don't think the church lasted very long."

A Book on the Train

Shortly before taking the train back to Augustana Seminary for his senior year, Granger bought a book that dramatically influenced his career. *The Art of Ministering to the Sick* had been published two years earlier in 1936.[8] The first author was Richard Clarke Cabot, a maverick physician who had practiced medicine at Massachusetts General Hospital and taught clinical medicine, social ethics, and philosophy at Harvard. Russell Dicks, the second author, was a Presbyterian minister and chaplain at Massachusetts General Hospital. Granger: "On the train I read all about the exciting things they were thinking and doing. In particular I was intrigued about the possibility of a physician and minister serving as a team in caring for people. It was a shame that I hadn't known about all of this during the time I was in Worcester."

Cabot and Dicks said that some doctors did not think that ministers could contribute to the care of hospitalized patients. In fact, the authors said some doctors worried that ministers would be a nuisance and might tire or excite patients. Cabot and Dicks argued that if the minister was prepared for his tasks, the minister indeed had important roles to play. They wrote: "The minister's opportunity in sickness is to devote himself to the growth of souls at a time when pain, sorrow, frustration and surprise, bring experiences that invite a new start in life."

The book described typical patients and the pain and opportunities they faced, the rituals of the sickroom, the roles of physicians, and institutional problems. It also provided practical advice regarding some ways ministers could be helpful to patients. This kind of information was not part of seminary curricula. In fact, Dicks later indicated that he and Cabot wrote the book for the following reason:[9] "There was not a single book or article upon the subject of ministering to the sick that had been written in this century. The last book that we could find was one published in England in the past century, whose thesis was that the minister's task in the sickroom was to prepare the sick person for death. There was no accepted precedent to follow and no recognized practice."

Granger returned to Augustana Seminary for his final year. Helen, now back home, struggled with whether to return to teaching. She recalled, "One morning as I was sitting on the front steps of our home, the principal and one of the school children came to visit. The principal acknowledged that I had had a rough previous school year. He asked me if I would like to teach seventh grade where there was less bedlam. He also invited me to be his assistant, a position that enabled me to be out of the classroom for one-third of the time. I said that I could only return if they stopped spanking the children. He agreed."

Granger and Helen were grateful to live close to one another, even though they were both very busy. Granger: "The last year of seminary was an exciting time because we seminarians were thinking about what kind of a congregation would invite us to serve as their pastor. Most of us came back from our internship with a better understanding of people who are in trouble or are searching for something vital in their lives, so we approached our studies with more enthusiasm. Unfortunately, we again spent most of our time in lectures. I thought it would have been helpful to have had dialogs with professors about how our experiences related to the subjects we were studying."

Granger's decision to become a Lutheran clergyman had major

implications for Helen. She was happy in the progressive First Presbyterian Church of Davenport that she had attended all her life. She taught in the church's religious education program that incorporated some of the latest understandings of how children learn. The program was so well regarded that seminarians from Augustana visited it. Helen and Granger were both fond of Helen's pastor, Dr. Alfred Nickless, a personable, well-educated man.

Helen was far less at home in the more conservative Lutheran church. Yet, as a future minister's wife, she was expected to take courses and become a Lutheran, steps she took willingly. Years later P. O. Bersell, the president of the Augustana Synod, asked Helen if she had become a Lutheran by "conviction" or "convenience." Helen: "I answered, 'convenience,' because I came from a wonderful church. Our conversation was in a pleasant tone, but he meant it, and I meant it."

Chapter 4

Ringing Church Bells

First English Lutheran Church of Bloomington, Illinois, was deeply in debt. Established in 1872 by about 60 Swedish immigrants, the church had grown and prospered. In 1923, English, rather than Swedish, became the official language of the church services. Four years later, the congregation built a lovely English Tudor style church and parsonage.

Not long after the new structures were built, the small, predominantly agricultural community of Bloomington was hit badly by the Depression. The church went into a decline. In 1938 the pastor became ill and had to resign. Few people attended services on Sunday morning, and the mortgage company was preparing to foreclose on the church's $30,000 loan.

In hopes of rebuilding their congregation, members of First English asked Conrad Bergendoff, then president of Augustana College and Theological Seminary, to propose three young candidates. Granger and two other seminarians each visited the church. Granger enjoyed challenges and was glad to be chosen as the new pastor.

Shortly after First English invited Granger to be their minister, but before he arrived to begin serving, the mortgage company announced that the church was to be put on the auction block. The church council members phoned Granger, who was still in the seminary, and asked him to join them ahead of schedule. Granger drove to Bloomington and helped the group that had gathered to pack the church valuables into a truck. Then, with tearful members watching, they solemnly drove the truck to the lawn of the McLean County Courthouse, where about 200 people had gathered for the auction.

When the bidding started, Granger bid $25,000 on behalf of the church, as he had been told to do. The bid, however, was unsuccessful. Officers of the mortgage company decided they had to keep the church, but they felt badly about the situation, so they asked Granger and the board members to meet privately with them. According to Granger, they said, "We're sorry about this. We don't know what we'll do with the church. We don't want you to start your ministry this way. Isn't there something you can do? We'll give you one more month if you think you can raise $5,000 more."

The grateful members of First English returned the truck to the church and unloaded the furniture and other valuables back into the building. The next day Granger led the Sunday morning service. With deeper feeling than usual, the congregation sang the old familiar hymn, "My Church, My Church, My Dear Old Church." Shortly after that, through the diligent efforts of the president of the Illinois Conference, the Lutheran Brotherhood Insurance Company took a first mortgage on the property totaling $20,000, and the Illinois Conference took a second mortgage for $8,000. A program was worked out so that the church could repay its debts in manageable monthly payments.

The effects of many lean years on First English were evident in the condition of the church and parsonage, which needed repairs and repainting. In celebration of the refinancing, church members pitched in, doing the work themselves. Granger returned to Augustana to complete his seminary education.

Ordination, the ceremony in which graduates of the seminary were admitted into the ministry, was held each year in conjunction with the annual meeting of the Augustana Lutheran Synod. The ordination for Granger's class of 1939 was held June 18 in Lindsborg,

Kansas. Because it was expensive to travel and Granger and Helen's wedding was two days later in Chicago, Granger's sister Lael was the only family member who attended the ordination.

It was customary on the day before the service of ordination for the president of the synod to question the candidates about their faith in front of a gathering of ministers. Granger:

> I was the last one. The 300 or so clergy in the audience were getting a bit weary. The question put to me by the president of the Augustana Synod, P. O. Bersell[1] was: "Mr. Westberg, we know your mother. She was very active in the church. I suppose that she encouraged you to be a minister."
>
> I suspected that Pastor Bersell was confusing my mother with our relative Corrine Westberg, who was a very active laywoman, but I answered him. "No, my mother didn't encourage me to go into the ministry. In fact she wanted to make it very difficult for me to go into the ministry."
>
> "Well," said Pastor Bersell, "If your mother doesn't think you should be in ministry, why should we think you should?" With this, the clergy broke into laughter. Then one of the prominent ministers rose and said, "I object to that kind of questioning." I responded, "The reason my mother didn't encourage me to go into the ministry is that it is such a high calling. She felt that it had to be my calling, not hers."

After his ordination service, Granger raced to Chicago for his wedding. Granger and Helen had planned to be married in her church in Davenport, but to accommodate his mother, Granger and Helen had a simple wedding in Chicago with only the immediate family in attendance. Helen's parents, her two sisters, and her maid of honor traveled from Davenport to Chicago. Helen's beloved Granna was too frail to make the trip. Granger and Helen were married by C. Emil Bergquist, Granger's pastor, and O. V. Anderson, their college professor and good friend. In the wedding picture, Helen looks lovely;

Granger is very thin. Eight years of putting himself through college and seminary, with only occasional full meals, had taken its toll.

Since Helen and Granger had only $75 between them, their options for a honeymoon were limited. For $15 they were able to stay at a cottage near Camp Augustana at Lake Geneva. With his summer work at Lake Geneva, the area had become important to Granger. Lake Geneva was also special for Helen, whose parents had spent time at the lake at the turn of the century.

Granger couldn't wait to get to his new church, so he and Helen cut short their honeymoon and headed to Bloomington. Granger: "The congregation had a huge debt, so we went to work. Every Sunday there were red envelopes in the pews for people to use in making their gifts of money. The people worked their heads off to pay down the debt."

By Christmas the church was turning around. The adult choir and the newly formed children's choir sang carols and anthems at the Christmas service. Traditionally the offering collected at this service was given to the pastor. Although Helen and Granger had very little income, they decided that the offering should be used to help pay off the church's debt. Upon hearing of Helen and Granger's generosity, the congregation also made substantial contributions.

On January 9, 1940, six months after Granger and Helen arrived at First English, an article appeared in the *Daily Pantograph*, the local Bloomington paper, with the headline: "Burdened Church Surges Ahead with Young Pastor's Leadership: But Rev. Westberg Would Credit Others." Reporter John Bowman wrote:

> If church people were like football fans and selected the minister who in their opinion did the most outstanding job of the last year, the Rev. Granger E. Westberg of English Lutheran Church surely would be one of the nominees. For in just six months since he took over the local pastorate, this handsome church has been changed from a dwindling organization discouraged

by heavy financial burdens to a lively, rapidly growing body
... Attendance has tripled and 23 new members were added to
the roster. The main room, which seats approximately 300,
was filled at several services. A new men's brotherhood class
was organized.

Modest yet inspiring with his frank, energetic manner, Mr.
Westberg is reluctant to take much credit for the progress. The
wiry, blonde, bespectacled young man says, "Anyone could
have done just as well with such a fine congregation. All they
needed was someone to suggest things to do. Virtually every
member helped tirelessly. It's amazing how unselfishly some
have been about stopping at the church before and after work
to help on various projects. It's very gratifying too, the amount
of self-sacrifice among members who were anxious to put a
big dent in the church debt by increasing their yearly pledges.
Some even put off buying new cars for another year."

One year after Granger began serving First English, a motion
was made at the annual meeting that Granger's salary be raised
from $1,600 to $1,700.[2] Granger: "After the motion was defeated, the
chairman of the board of trustees explained to others, 'Granger is a
new pastor. He's done a good job, but I don't think we should overdo it.'"

This chairman of the board was also the superintendent of the
Sunday school. At the end of each Sunday school session, Granger
and Helen would have to contain themselves when the superintendent
said, "Let us say the Lord's Prayer responsively, and then all pass out."

An Ecumenical Spirit

With his ecumenical leanings, Granger was eager to get acquainted
with other pastors and churches in Bloomington. The nearby Lutheran
church was part of the Missouri Lutheran Synod. Missouri Lutherans
did not regard members of other Lutheran groups as true Lutherans.
They offered communion only to members of their synod. Lutheran

ministers from other synods were not invited to preach from Missouri pulpits.

Early one Sunday morning, before his own service, Granger slipped into the back row of the Missouri Synod church, just as members of the congregation were preparing for their early service. No one recognized Granger because he was not wearing his clerical collar and he was new in the community. Suddenly the janitor hurried into the back of the church. In German he pleaded for someone to help him ring the large bell. Granger's high school German paid off. Eagerly, he volunteered and followed the janitor up into the bell tower. The largest bell was so heavy that it required two strong people to start it moving. The janitor held the bell's rope, while standing on a rise. When Granger pushed the bell, the janitor swung off the riser, using all of his weight to ring the bell.

Later, someone discovered it was Granger who had helped with the bell and that he was a minister. Soon the story spread through the town. The janitor was upset to learn that he had asked a pastor to help him with the bell.

The next night, the janitor came to the Westberg parsonage with his straw hat in his hands. He apologized profusely, while polishing the sweaty headband from his hat with his handkerchief. Granger and Helen assured the man that there was no problem. Granger said that he had been happy to help.

Not long after that, Granger was surprised one morning to see the pastor of the Missouri Synod church at the door of the parsonage. Granger: "The pastor said, 'I'm sorry this happened.' 'Sorry?' I said, 'I enjoyed it.' 'Well, I just want you to know,' the pastor said, 'that this is the first time I've ever visited another Protestant minister who isn't Missouri Synod.' Granger invited the pastor into the parsonage and church. The pastor declined to enter the church, but he did go into the parsonage. During Granger and Helen's tenure in Bloomington, the minister never entered First English Church, despite other invitations from Granger.

Granger found much more openness among the Presbyterians. Granger recalled, "I was fond of Harold Martin, pastor of the local Presbyterian church. He showed me around his church and introduced me to the choir director, a young woman who had a magic touch with children. There were 100 people in her several choirs. Some months later, they sang at our church. Later Harold became moderator of the nationwide Presbyterian Church of America."

The years 1939 through 1958 were the era of Pope Pius XII in the Roman Catholic Church. Being Catholic meant going to church every Sunday, not eating meat on Friday, fasting during Lent, praying with a rosary, and saying confession to a priest in a confessional booth. Priests said Mass in Latin. Most parishioners did not raise questions or challenge the authority of the church or the pope. Protestants and Roman Catholics had many misconceptions about each other.

In the late 1930s there was little or no official contact between Roman Catholic and Lutheran clergy. Granger, however, was interested in meeting his Catholic counterparts and learning more about the Roman Catholic Church:

> There was a Roman Catholic church about two blocks from our church. I heard they had a young priest, so I went there and rang the bell of the rectory. Father Jerome turned out to be my age. He was a warm-hearted man from the order of St. Francis—the poorest priests of all. It was a very hot day, so, after we talked for a while, I asked him how he could wear such a heavy cassock. He replied by quickly pulling up his cassock and revealing a pair of red-hot shorts.
>
> Father Jerome invited me to bring my confirmation class to his church, so I brought about 12 youngsters. While we were there, he gave us a play-by-play account of the Mass. When the children went home, they told their parents about our visit with Father Jerome at his church. They also apparently indicated that I had said positive things about Catholics, including the

fact that they too are Christians. A couple of parents were very upset that I talked so positively about Catholics.

I invited Father Jerome to bring his class to our church. He said, "I'd like to do that, but at this time the road only leads in one direction." Forty years later when I was speaking to clergy in New Orleans, Father Jerome came up and introduced himself. I learned that he had been working with people with Hansen's disease [leprosy]. What a dedicated guy."

When Granger was invited to write an article for *The Lutheran Companion*, he chose to write about the strategies for ecumenism that he was introducing to his confirmands. He wrote: "Lutheran youth must learn to join hands with all Christians. A most profitable evening could be spent together with the leader of another church group. After the formal talk, 'pepper' that person with questions. Find out how in your own local community you might put on a united program of Christian service."

When Granger received the edition of the journal in which his article was printed, he was upset to discover that this and other statements he had written had been omitted. In their place were excerpts from a Bible story and some rather syrupy recommendations for leading a devout life. His manuscript had been rewritten without his knowledge or permission.

In addition to introducing the confirmation class to Roman Catholicism, Granger worked with them on the usual subjects addressed in the year prior to confirmation. However, rather than having them mindlessly memorize the material, as he had to do as a confirmand, he encouraged them to question and to reflect on what they read and heard. He also introduced a topic that typically was not part of the traditional curriculum—human sexuality. With permission from the board of deacons, the confirmation class and a few parents spent three classes on "God's Gift of the Human Body," taught by a church member who was a physiologist.[3]

Alongside the existing educational programs for children and youth, Granger wanted programs for young adults. He thought that a good way to be in touch with at least some young adults would be to establish a branch of the Lutheran Student Association at Illinois State University. Granger convinced his Missouri Synod pastor neighbor and some other Lutheran pastors about the worthiness of doing this. They agreed, so Granger, the pastors, and some students set up a chapter of the association.

After Granger and his clergy colleagues made connections with students at the campus, many of the students started attending church services at First English, as well as the other Lutheran churches. Granger: "The students who came to our church included 25 young men, who before serving in the Navy V-12 program at Illinois State University had been attending Augustana College. Some of them had been members of the Augustana Choir and had good, well-trained voices. Many of them joined our choir, so before long, the choir had 25 men and 15 women. When the choir processed into the church singing a hymn, it was a thrilling experience."

Helen as Minister's Wife

As the minister's wife, Helen was expected to be actively involved in the life of the church, without a salary. Granger was proud of the work Helen did, including serving as a Girl Scouts counselor, being a member of three women's groups, and teaching Bible study. Helen also started a new group for young businesswomen called "the Deo Juvante Society" that had a threefold mission—devotions, mission study, and socializing. Over the years, they gathered clothing for the poor, gave gifts of food at Christmas, did sewing for the local hospitals, and organized the first annual Mother and Daughter Banquet.

Many of the church members who were farmers supplied Granger and Helen with fresh produce and eggs. A few even brought them freshly killed chickens. One woman invited Helen to her home and showed her how to pluck a chicken. Helen decided that the process of pulling out the feathers under scalding water was not for her. She declined further lessons.

Overall, Helen enjoyed her work. In her later years, she recalled: "I thought being a minister's wife was great. I intended to go on doing it, but that didn't happen."

Giving the Board a Cold Existential Experience

As Granger and Helen approached their second winter in Bloomington, they knew they had to find a way to keep their home warm. Granger: "Our parsonage was attractive in every way, except for the heating. It had no insulation in the ceiling or roof. Wind came through the windows of the living room, which was made still colder because of its cathedral ceilings. Our first winter, we couldn't use the living room because it was so cold. The second winter we were especially concerned because Helen was pregnant."

In those days the church owned and made all the decisions regarding the minister's home. That meant that Granger and Helen had to persuade the board of the church to authorize funds for insulating the parsonage. Granger:

> To help the board of trustees understand the problem, Helen and I decided we'd invite them to have their usual monthly meeting in our living room. It was a cold day in November. As the evening wore on, the chairman of the board whispered to me, "Do you have a fire in the furnace?" "Yes," I said. "Come see it." He and I went down into the basement. When I opened the furnace, he could see the roaring fire. He went upstairs, interrupted the meeting, and invited the others to go down into the basement and see the fire. Very soon funds were authorized for insulating the parsonage.

The more Granger involved himself deeply in the community, the more new themes for ministry emerged. At the time, ministers did not typically counsel with couples who were seeking to be married.

They simply discussed the logistics of the marriage ceremony. Granger was concerned about the growing number of divorces and felt that when he married a couple, he was responsible for ensuring that they were ready for marriage.

In 1941, Granger wrote an article in which he challenged the custom of ministers performing "on-the-spot marriages."[14] He recommended that ministers meet with the couple on two different occasions and discuss such issues as the length of their relationship, their knowledge of each other's backgrounds, and ideas for dealing with future problems. He wanted the couple to realize that the minister was interested in them and they could turn to him for help in the future.

Granger's concern about helping to promote strong marriages might have been linked to his becoming a father. In March 1941 Helen gave birth to their first child, Jane Christine, at a Roman Catholic hospital in Bloomington. Helen's physician prescribed the then usual 10 days of bed rest in the hospital. Granger visited Helen and Jane daily. Each evening, when visiting hours were over, the nuns asked Granger to stay and talk. They peppered him with questions about the Bible—a book that they were not encouraged to study.

Music, Music

Even though First English had a well-developed music program, Granger missed the majestic sound of a pipe organ in their church. First English had a little reed pump organ that was powered with a vacuum cleaner motor because it was too difficult for the organist to pump continuously while playing. The sound of the organ was thin and the volume weak.

One evening when Granger and Helen were at a movie theater, Granger spied the pipe organ that had been played during silent films. With some detective work he identified the owner, who was willing to sell it for a very low price. Granger found Fred Hunt, an organ builder, who said he could rebuild it for the church. With his enthusiasm, Granger convinced the congregation to go ahead with the project.

The project took 18 months to complete. Martha Rinker, a local reporter, wrote in Bloomington's, newspaper, *The Pantagraph*:

> Piece by piece the mighty Barton pipe organ, valued at more than $10,000, is being moved from the Majestic Theater ... No ordinary theater organ this, equipped mainly with bells and drums and cymbals, but a veritable symphony orchestra with pipes for violin, clarinet, flute, oboe and tuba.
>
> Almost the entire basement of the parish hall of the church was needed to store the thousands of parts ... The Rev. Granger Westberg has requested that the first dedicatory composition to be played be the *Toccata and Fugue in D Minor* by Bach, for he says, "This organ must immediately inherit the great Lutheran tradition of Bach and his church music."

The church was packed on the day the organ was dedicated. Granger: "We carefully arranged to open the service by having our organist, Ray Olson, play the little old pump organ. Then, as the little pump organ was performing poorly, Fred Hunt began playing Bach's *Toccata and Fugue in D Minor* on the organ he had newly restored, pulling out all the stops. Everyone was astounded. The powerful, rich sound of the pipe organ drowned out the old pump organ."

Helen: "Getting the organ assembled was a lot of work for everyone. On the day after the dedication, the president of the board, Fred Anderson, drove into our driveway. I said to him, 'Well, Fred, you can all relax now.' He shook his head and looked at me so pitifully. 'No,' he responded, 'Granger will think of something else.' How true that's been all through the years."

A Rousing Sermon

Amid building community connections and exploring new dimensions of ministry, Granger remained faithful to his calling as a preacher.

He worked hard on his sermons—sometimes with surprising results.[5]

> Early in my ministry I gave a rousing sermon entitled "Serve
> the Lord with Gladness." I wanted to stir up my people so that
> they would want to serve the Lord. My sermon dealt primarily
> with the usual vague generalities. In fact it was about as vague
> as it could be. But apparently the sermon moved two ladies
> in their early 40s to some action. They stopped me after the
> service and said that now that their children were away at
> school, they had some free time during the day. What did I
> suggest they do? I couldn't think of a thing. No one had taken
> my preaching quite so literally before.

Later in the week when Granger remembered that the local hospital
had closed one of its floors for lack of nursing staff, he suggested to
the women that they talk to the hospital administrator and see if they
could be of some help. In those days most hospitals were making
little or no use of volunteers. "The administrator wasn't the least bit
interested and told them that he could use only registered nurses.
Later he told me not to send any more 'do-gooders' over because the
hospital couldn't use these people. They would just be in the way."

The women, however, were not discouraged. Granger wrote:
"They got in touch with several of the nurses at the hospital, who put
pressure on the administrator, reminding him how shorthanded they
really were, arguing that they could think of many tasks volunteers
could do to relieve registered nurses."

The administrator reluctantly yielded, and the women began to
help in the hospital, doing such chores as making beds and feeding
children and elderly patients. "The two women found that it lifted
their spirits immensely to engage in what they saw to be a worthwhile
Christian service. They told me that life was actually brighter for them
now. Working in the hospital had forced them to forget themselves
and to think of others."

Granger was intrigued and excited by the fact that people wanted to give and that giving could have healthy benefits for those who gave.

More than Preaching

Although Granger wanted to be an effective preacher, he was becoming increasingly convinced that one of a pastor's most important roles might be as a counselor.[6] In the seminary, Granger and his classmates had been taught to make house calls on parishioners and potential new church members, visit them in the hospital, and teach them through sermons and other means. Granger felt that most of these kinds of interactions were superficial.

He remembered his helpful conversations with Pastor Bergquist. He knew that psychiatry and clinical psychology emphasized the importance of listening to people and supporting them in their struggles, and he knew that a growing number of people were going to these professionals for counseling. Granger felt that the clergy could also provide some kind of counseling.

Granger was eager to have serious conversations with members of his congregation. But weeks went by without Granger seeing parishioners for "personal interviews." One summer, in an attempt to determine if this was also a problem in other parishes, Granger put the following question in a questionnaire that he and his colleagues distributed to young people attending Camp Augustana: "How many times a year do you have a private conversation with your pastor?" When most of the youth responded, "Never," Granger and his colleagues followed up by asking the young people why this was true. The reason most often given was: "I've never had any serious problems to talk to him about. Why should I bother him?"

In response, Granger wrote:[7] "It is true that a doctor or lawyer is seldom consulted unless there is a special reason, but shouldn't a clergyman be thought of as one who specializes more in preventive therapy than in crisis therapy?"

To start the ball rolling on his plan to engage his congregation in serious conversation, including counseling, Granger sent postcards to adult and youth members of in the church, inviting them to meet with him in his church study alone or with a friend. After each conversation, Granger tried to spend five minutes recording the key information and issues that had emerged: "I wasn't doing anything fancy. I felt that just as doctors and nurses took time to write down what they had learned from patients that I also should write down and reflect on what I had learned."

This practice of making notes, however brief, after each pastoral encounter put Granger on a trajectory that would take him out of the parish, although never out of the church.

Chapter 5

Thrown to the Wolves

In 1941, two years after Granger had begun his ministry in Bloomington, Illinois, he underwent a life-changing series of events that were to have an enormous impact on his career. Granger and some other young clergymen were eating lunch together at a ministerial conference in Chicago when a pastor in his 80s asked if he could join them. The elderly pastor turned out to be the part-time chaplain of Augustana Lutheran Hospital, an institution Granger knew well because his father's company helped build the hospital when Granger was a boy.

In response to questions from Granger and others, Chaplain Carl Christenson regaled the group with stories about the trials and tribulations of ministering to a hospital full of sick people. Midway through the meal, in a comment that was meant to be facetious, he said, "I have to be away for a week next month. Would any of you young men be interested in taking my place?"

Granger: "I found myself volunteering to do that. Chaplain Christenson then went on to say, 'Well, Granger, you should know that the doctors and nurses will be surprised to see a young fellow like you taking my place. After all the average age of hospital chaplains is 77, or they have heart trouble and need to be close to medical help.'"

When Christenson saw that Granger was serious, he made arrangements for Granger to take over his duties for a week and to stay in the medical interns' quarters. A month later, Granger arrived at Augustana Hospital to begin his week of work. He found a note from Chaplain Christenson welcoming him and instructing him to visit every patient every day. Granger: "The hospital had eight floors and 300 beds. I tried all that morning to do as I was told, but by noon I couldn't continue running from room to room, greeting people. I felt more like a hostess than a chaplain."

At lunchtime, Granger went down to the dining room, where he thought he would sit with the doctors. As he headed toward a table of doctors, the person in charge of the dining room intercepted him and explained that the chaplain always sat at the administrators' table. Granger:

It happened that the auditors were there that week, so all that the administrators talked about was dollars and cents, which was of little interest to me.

I could overhear a group of doctors at the next table talking about patients. Later in the day I asked the top administrator, E. I. Erikson, if it would be all right for me to sit at one of the doctor's tables for the rest of the week. "No," he replied, "I think you'd better not. The chaplain has sat at this table for 50 years." When I pressed him, he shook his head and said, "I'm afraid the doctors wouldn't care to have a clergyman at their table." He hesitated. "You see, their language isn't always the best." When I assured him that I had heard a few rather expressive words in my life and could probably stand it for a week, he finally agreed I might try it, but he was sure the doctors wouldn't be pleased. It was as if he were throwing me to the wolves. I soon found out he was not far from right.

After lunch I went back on the floors determined not to run from bed to bed welcoming folks, so I looked for the friendliest nurse I could find and told her that I was pinch-hitting for the chaplain and that I'd like her to find the people who really needed what I had to give. Her reply was, "What is it you have to give?" Then she caught herself and said, "I don't mean to be disrespectful, but we have a lot of preachers coming here every day preaching at people. Do you preach at people?" I said I hoped I didn't preach. I said the Lord gave us two ears and one mouth so that we should listen twice as much as we talk. I hoped I listened to what people were thinking about. That made her feel more comfortable. She continued, "Do you pray over people?" I replied, "I hope I don't pray over people. I pray with them. If I have a prayer it's because the patient seems ready for it."

The nurse then told me that there was a patient who might like to talk with me. He had two teenagers who were driving him nuts. The nurse asked the man, and he agreed that I could visit him. Right away he started telling me about his problems. After a short time he said something like, "You know, chaplain. I've done more serious thinking in the last few days in the hospital that I have done for many months, even years." That was a theme that I was to hear all week long.

At the next meal, dressed in my clerical attire, I sat at one of the doctors' tables. A young resident turned to me and in a semi-friendly way said, 'What in the _____ are you doing here at this table?' I explained that I was there for a week to see how the church carried on its ministry of healing. Startled, he said, "Church? Its ministry of healing? The doctors do all the healing around here. The church just hires some tired old man to pass out tracts." Later in the conversation the resident continued, "I know the church has done a good job with buildings, equipment, and beds, but why doesn't it get more interested in doing something for the patients as people?"

For the remainder of the week I got less sleep and drank more coffee than during any other week of my life. I went on every emergency call, and as I would walk back to the interns' quarters with a young doctor, he would say things like, "I sewed up a wound. What did you do, chaplain?" Then I would try to describe the talk I had had with the father of a teenage boy who had been injured in an auto accident. I told him how the father had blamed himself for the fact that his son associated with a gang of hoodlums who drove around town in search of excitement. In his introspective mood, the father admitted that he had never gone out of his way to develop a close relationship with his son. He said that just seeing a clergyman reminded him of how he had erred in this way. He hoped he might have another chance to prove that he could be a better father.

This kind of discussion went on all week. It seemed that the hospital was alive with frightened people who had been stopped in their tracks for the first time in many years. They wanted to talk with someone who represented a power greater than themselves. Here was a concentration of anxious, worried people, figuratively begging for someone to take a personal interest in them. During that one week, I saw more people who wanted to talk about vital matters than I had found in my church in several months.

When this exciting week ended, I had the feeling that more serious thinking was taking place per square foot in a hospital than in any other building in the community, including the nearby college. I was able to minister to patients effectively in a very short time because when people are lying horizontally in a hospital, they begin to think about the vertical dimension of life. They wonder about the meaning of life and start asking spiritual questions. But there's usually no one around to help them deal with those difficult questions, so they don't get very far with their thinking.

I was also sure that if the church felt the Christian faith had anything to say to people in time of trouble, the best place to have its pastor say it was in the context of suffering, anxiety, birth and death. Where else could a minister find people so ready to talk about spiritual concerns?

A Life Shift

This was the era in which patients typically stayed in the hospital for a week or more, so there was, indeed, time for them to be reflective. Granger said, "When I returned home, I could scarcely think of anything but the church's opportunity for bringing words of faith and hope through its ministry in its scores of outstanding hospitals. I sensed that there were tremendous opportunities in the hospital setting where people were asking essentially theological questions which related to the meaning of life."

Granger shared his ideas with Chaplain Christenson and E. I. Erickson, the hospital administrator. Granger was 27 and had worked as a chaplain for only one week. The men were his elders. But that didn't stop him.

Granger complimented Chaplain Christenson on his work but pointed out that even an efficient chaplain could not be expected to handle the volume of work connected with a hospital the size of Augustana. Granger recommended hiring one or more pastoral intern assistants so that a clergy person could be on duty at all times. Having assistants, argued Granger, would "give visible evidence of the importance of spiritual care; cause our nurses to see that the services of clergymen and doctors are of equal importance;" and allow the regular chaplain to do more counseling with patients, nurses, and family members.

Granger also said there was an acute need for a chapel and for religious artwork and listed other needs and problems as well as possible solutions.

Granger then sent a letter full of ideas to the board of trustees at the hospital. Apparently they were not too put off with cocky, young Granger because soon they sent him a letter appointing him to a committee charged with developing ideas for the chaplaincy department at the hospital.

Weeks later the committee met with Chaplain Christenson to get acquainted with him and his work. Granger said that when they asked Chaplain Christenson how they could support him, he responded, "I would like the privilege of no longer having to fill out a statistical report indicating the number of people I've seen or the amount of literature I've passed out. I'd like to feel free to stop at the bedside of those people who I feel I can help. Doing this means some people who come into the hospital may never have a visit from the chaplain. But I'm not sure every patient needs a visit."

The committee unanimously adopted Chaplain Christenson's suggestions.

Granger's experience at Augustana Hospital helped him think even more deeply about his ministry to his Bloomington parishioners who were ill. He was eager to find some way that he and his parishioners' physicians could work together. Years later in his book *Minister and Doctor Meet*[1] he reflected on his experience in the parish:

> It was my plan that when any of my parishioners became ill,
> I would go to his or her physician and offer my services in a
> 'team approach' to illness. Since no one had ever spelled it out
> for me, I wasn't exactly sure what this team was to do. But I had
> a vague feeling that somehow the physician and the minister
> belonged together.
>
> When a parishioner went to the hospital a few days after I
> was installed in my first parish, I called her doctor. As nearly
> as I can remember, the conversation went something like this:
> "Dr. Smith? One of my parishioners, Mrs. Johnson, is your
> patient and before I go to the hospital to call on her, I wonder
> if there is anything you think I might be able to do that would
> be of help." There was a long silence at the other end of the line.

When Dr. Smith had caught his breath, he said: "Well, ah ... I don't know anything about your business, Reverend. I make it a point to keep off the subject of religion. I can't tell you how to run your affairs." This pretty well finished the conversation, and I knew there would be no point in calling him again.

When a second parishioner became ill, Granger summoned his courage and made a personal call at the doctor's office. Unable to understand the purpose of his call, the receptionist listed Granger as a new patient. The doctor gave him a warm welcome, but when Granger told him his mission, the doctor said, "Oh, I can't think of anything in particular you can do for Mrs. Bland. Just pray for her. Everybody can stand a prayer now and then, don't you think?"

Granger could sense that the interview was over. It bothered him to think that when his people were sick, he wasn't considered a member of the healing team. Granger: "It didn't seem right to me that the physician and the minister should be miles apart in their thinking when they spent so much time in hospitals dealing with the same people. The thought kept occurring to me that maybe doctors and ministers ought to get acquainted on a professional level. Unfortunately, I hadn't the slightest notion of how to go about this."

Granger wrote that he remembered that when he first read "the exciting description of new ways of ministering to people under stress" in the Cabot and Dick's book, *The Art of Ministering to the Sick*, he "was led to contemplate a team approach to the care of my parishioners." Now, he had to admit that he wasn't being very successful in doing this. Perhaps, he thought, he had better step back and clarify his own role in ministering to the sick before proposing to collaborate with a physician.

Granger decided that he needed to take the advice of Dicks and Cabot and reflect deeply on his conversations with patients by taking notes on his interactions with patients that were more detailed than the notes he took after meeting with members of his parish who visited him in his office.

In their book, Dicks and Cabot argued that deeply reflective note-taking would enable ministers to clarify the process, check their understanding, identify what they needed to do next, and learn how to enhance their own effectiveness. Granger wrote that he decided to write down as much of the conversation as he could remember and then ask himself such questions as:[2]

- Was this a patient-centered call or did I take over and talk about myself?
- After calling on the patient, do I know more about him or her?
- What were the themes of our discussion, and why did the patient choose these themes?
- How does the patient perceive me and how do I plan to help him or her? In other words, why am I spending time with this person?

After Granger pinch-hit for the chaplain of Augustana Hospital in 1941, he was in regular communication with the hospital as a member of the committee for Christian activities. His article titled, "Are Church Hospitals Different?," which was published in January 1943, shows that he was giving a great deal of thought to the role of church hospitals.[3]

The Protestant church has done a great work in building hospitals in our country. Many communities would be without hospitals had not leading Protestant clergymen and laymen taken the matter in hand, raised funds from out of the churches, and erected institutions that today are serving the medical profession in an excellent manner. However, were these Protestant hospitals organized solely for the purpose of serving the medical man—to give him a building in which to do his work? Or was there also a religious purpose in establishing them?

Whatever the situation in those days, it is becoming

increasingly clear that if we as a Lutheran church are to stay in the "hospital business," we must restudy and re-examine our reasons for wanting to do so.

Granger argued that to create good will, the heritage of Protestant hospitals should be reflected in the hospital's name, in pictures and furnishings, and in a chapel that would be "the center of the hospital's life" through its daily services for staff, patients, and family members. Further, there should be a full-time chaplain—a rarity at that time. If that was not possible, a local parish pastor could coordinate the visits of local pastors so that the same pastor could give continuity of care to the patients assigned to him.

Speaking in the male gendered language of his time, Granger said that the ideal chaplain who would work in these Protestant hospitals would have a year of preparation for his work. For example, he might work as an assistant to a skillful chaplain, such as Dr. Otis Rice, chaplain of St. Luke's Hospital in New York City. While on the hospital staff, the trainee would be given opportunities to work as a "male nurse" so he could see operations first hand. In addition, Granger recommended that the trainee take courses in psychology.

Granger clearly understood the importance of collaborating with others while building new programs. He wrote that when beginning his new work, the ideal chaplain should work closely with the medical staff. If the staff is involved in planning the "religious program," Granger said, they would probably have a "keener interest in it."

Granger also wrote that it was important for the chaplain to earn the respect of the nursing staff. The chaplain could do this in part by offering a course for nurses that included discussions of pastoral psychology and how the chaplain could contribute to the care of the patient. If the chaplain does not gain the nurses' support, Granger warned, he will begin his work with "two strikes against him." On the other hand, nurses can help "pave the way for the entry of the chaplain into a room of a difficult patient." Also, nurses can "be especially helpful in recommending that the chaplain see certain patients and, in advance, give him helpful hints from her observation of the person."

Granger thought the chaplain should have a private office where he could counsel doctors, nurses, other clergy, and the relatives of patients. The chaplain should also have a portable communion set and other equipment that would enable him to minister in patients' rooms. Further, there should be portable headsets for patients so they could listen to services and recorded music. In general, Granger envisioned the ideal chaplain as being "on par with the medical staff—where spiritual therapy was given as much consideration as physical therapy."

Granger's article on church hospitals was well received by a number of people in the emerging field of pastoral care, including, Seward Hiltner, who was then executive secretary of the Commission on Religion and Health of the Federal Council of the Churches of Christ in America. Hiltner, who met Granger in the summer of 1942, wrote to Dan Williams, Granger's brother-in-law, telling him he liked Granger's article and he was "enormously impressed" with Granger. "I hope I shall be able to keep in touch with him and that eventually he will get full time into the hospital ministry, as I think he has a real aptitude for it."

Granger's thinking about the ideal chaplain continued to evolve. In early 1943, he wrote that the chaplain had four major tasks:[4]

1. Working with individual patients.
2. Counseling with relatives.
3. Giving lectures and providing conferences to nurses and doctors.
4. Conducting intensive pastoral clinics for students and pastors and lecturing on "religion and health."

In the same article, in a day when little attention was given to prevention and much attention was placed on "wonder drugs" and technology, Granger reiterated what was becoming a major theme for him. Even at this early stage in his chaplaincy work, he recognized that parish pastors were on the front line. "Parish pastors have easy and natural access to people, putting them in a unique position for being counselors who can help prevent illness and who can detect early stages of illness and direct people to appropriate help."

A Pioneering Possibility

In 1943 Chaplain Christenson became very ill and had to retire. "Our committee was asked to select 'a young man in his late 60s or early 70s,'" Granger joked.

> Actually, we approached a number of clergy in their 50s and 60s. All of them were insulted to be considered for this position because they thought it implied that we thought they were ready for retirement or that maybe they were doing an inadequate job in their parish and should therefore take a less demanding hospital position.
>
> As I sought to persuade each candidate to consider the position seriously, I was, in effect, talking to myself. When one person after another turned down the position, I came to realize that this field of service was very misunderstood. Why should this work be limited to older men? Wouldn't the hospital offer a challenge to a younger man?
>
> By exclusively hiring retired clergy, the hospital was indicating only a token interest in the religious dimensions of the healing ministry. As long as the hospital had a chaplain, it fulfilled the letter of the law. When these older men had new ideas or suggestions, they were often told that their jobs were only temporary and, therefore, they shouldn't begin a project they might not be around to complete.

The committee received one refusal after another. They wondered where to turn next. Granger was so bothered by the situation that one day in a committee meeting he blurted out, "Have you ever thought of me?" Obviously they had not, and they considered his proposal to be humorous indeed. It took him a long time to convince them he was serious. But they finally called him to be the new chaplain of Augustana Hospital.

Chapter 6

Verbatim

Granger was called as a full-time, not a part-time, chaplain. This was a big step for a Protestant hospital. In 1940 a commission of the American Protestant Hospitals Association, headed by Russell Dicks, surveyed its 400 Protestant hospitals. Only 18 of the 214 responding hospitals had full-time chaplains. The low regard in which chaplains were held was reflected in their inadequate salaries. Thirty percent were paid less than $1,000 a year. Only three received salaries commensurate with the average clergy person. In many of the hospitals, administrators, who were themselves clergy, acted as chaplains.[1] In contrast, Roman Catholic hospitals typically had ordained chaplains.[2]

Granger saw enormous potential for hospital chaplains. Inspired by the work of Dicks and others, he resolved to help reshape hospital chaplaincy and to raise the level of professionalism in the field. He was personally eager to learn about the contributions that psychology and psychiatry were making to pastoral care. In his letter of resignation from First English Lutheran Church, Granger said that although he would not begin serving as chaplain until the fall of 1944, he wanted to leave early so he could begin to prepare himself for his new work.

In an article in the *Daily Pantograph,* announcing that Granger was leaving the parish for a hospital post, it's clear that Granger's plans for education in pastoral care extended beyond himself. He was already thinking of Augustana Hospital as a future site for the clinical education of clergy, a concept that was still very new. In the *Daily Pantagraph* article, he is quoted as saying, "In view of the increasing demand upon pastors to be specifically trained in the field of pastoral psychology and psychiatry, the need has long been felt for a clinical training center to which theological students could go as pastoral interns to receive the practical experience of work with patients in a hospital."

O. V. Anderson, Granger's former professor who chaired one of Augustana Hospital's boards, was pleased with Granger's enthusiasm. However, as a former businessman who understood how resistant most organizations are to change, he was concerned that Granger was moving too quickly. In a supportive letter to Granger,[3] O. V. commended him for his good ideas but cautioned him about talking publicly about building a chapel and having a training program for theological students and pastors at Augustana. "To some people," O. V. wrote, "Your ideas will sound too big and too novel. If a few disgruntled individuals start a whispering campaign, you will have two strikes on you before you get up to bat."

Changes in His Personal Life

On February 7, 1944, Granger and Helen's second child, John Granger, was born. After John's birth, Granger made many trips into Chicago to make arrangements for his new work and his pre-work education. He also found a temporary home for the family—an apartment above a church on the south side of Chicago.

Meanwhile Helen had to pack and to manage John and Jane, largely without Granger's help. This pattern of Helen shouldering the responsibility of the home front while Granger was away pursuing projects continued even after she and Granger had four children.

Later, speaking of the time in the temporary third floor home where there was no elevator and the family had to be quiet because of the church below, Granger admitted: "These were busy, difficult, and lonely months for Helen. The apartment was only partly furnished, and she had the full care of our two youngsters. She was a good sport."

Although a few young pioneers were now working as Protestant hospital chaplains, most of the public still considered it an area of work for old men. Granger: "My decision to become a hospital chaplain was perhaps hardest on my mother. For fully five years after I became a chaplain, she said that people would say to her, 'Mrs. Westberg, what happened to your boy?' or 'Mrs. Westberg, will Granger get a real church again some day?' One pastor solemnly grasped her hand and said, 'I'm so sorry to hear that your son has left the ministry.'"

Preparing Himself

When Granger thought through how to prepare himself to be a chaplain (and how to prepare others to provide pastoral care to members of their congregations), he saw enticing possibilities. Because of the pioneering efforts of physicians Richard Cabot and Helen Flanders Dunbar and clergy, including Russell Dicks, Anton Boisen, and August Philip Guiles, a few general and mental hospitals were offering clinical training in which clergy and seminarians could interact to varying degrees with patients and reflect on their experiences with clinical supervisors.

Granger consulted with Lael's husband, Dan Williams, who, in 1939 had joined the faculty of Chicago Theological Seminary as a professor of contemporary theology. Dan counseled Granger to take courses at the University of Chicago, saying that the department of practical theology was eager to prepare clergy for the kind of work Granger wanted to do.

Granger also conferred with Russell Dicks. Dicks, who had been chaplain at Massachusetts General from 1932 to 1939, where he worked with Dr. Cabot, now lived in Dallas. He wrote Granger that he was moving from Dallas to Wesley Hospital in Chicago. "It is my plan," he said, "to set up an informal course there for clergymen who desire training in the general pastoral work field. I am sure it would be possible for me to give you some special attention in your work at Augustana [Hospital]." He also recommended that Granger spend time with two clergy pioneers: Rollin Fairbanks at Massachusetts General Hospital and August Phillip Guiles at Boston City Hospital.[4]

After consulting also with other leaders in the new field, Granger proposed to the board of directors at Augustana Hospital that he spend six months preparing for his new work. In the spring, he would begin with courses at the University of Chicago that would provide him with a theoretical groundwork. He would also study with Russell Dicks. During the summer he would do clinical pastoral education with Anton Boisen at Elgin State Hospital (a "mental hospital") and at Massachusetts General Hospital. This would give him a taste of the two approaches to clinical education—a more psychoanalytic approach at Elgin and a more pastoral care approach at Massachussetts General. Granger proposed that he would return to Chicago for more work with Dicks. The Augustana Hospital board liked the proposal and agreed to pay for Granger's courses and housing.

Granger enjoyed his class work at the University of Chicago and was stimulated by the presence of bright theologians and students from many denominations. He especially appreciated the opportunity to sit in on classes taught by Dan Williams, "my favorite theologian." However, the classes Granger took with Russell Dicks, who taught at Northwestern (Garrett Evangelical Theological Seminary) were even more on target. Dicks also personally worked with Granger at Wesley Hospital over a four-month period.

Granger: "Dicks fascinated us by scrutinizing every word spoken by pastors in sick rooms. He wrote the verbatim on the left hand side of the paper. On the right side of the page, he wrote comments about and critique of the conversation. When he was out of town I taught his classes.

"What a break it was for me to work closely with the clergyman who helped start the whole idea of a professional chaplaincy. We each began our separate chaplaincy programs in Chicago; he at Wesley Memorial Hospital (now Northwestern University Hospital) and I at Augustana Lutheran Hospital." Both hospitals were on the near north side of Chicago, about a mile and a half apart.

After studying with Dicks, Granger participated in Anton Boisen's program at Elgin State Hospital, a "mental hospital" for emotionally troubled people. In those days general and mental hospitals typically were separate. People with a wide range of mental health problems were removed from society into hospitals like Elgin State. This was before the advent of effective anti-psychotic medications. Patients were heavily sedated. Some wore straight jackets.

Granger said that Boisen was a very revered figure with a great deal of credibility because he had been a patient in a mental hospital. His autobiography, *Exploration of the Inner Life*,[5] was based on some of the letters Boisen had written to Lael's boss, Fred Eastman, a professor at Chicago Theological Seminary, during his emotional struggles. Granger recalled, "Boisen had a warm spirit and a soft voice. Often he was quiet. Although he wasn't an openly demonstrative person, he was loving in his own way. He was an advocate for more research into ways of dealing with the spiritual needs of mental patients."

Boisen was convinced that some psychotic episodes were people's efforts to reorganize and heal their souls, so he thought that students of pastoral care needed to work to understand what was happening. He also felt that the church had something to offer to the patients. Boisen saw the hospital in Elgin as a kind of laboratory in which students, under supervision, could learn from the "living human document."

Granger recalled:

The other students and I spent our time visiting patients, writing up cases, and then discussing them with Boisen and each other. I found that I was comfortable in this setting, essentially because most of our pastoral care work in this hospital was done in the presence of helpful nurses and doctors who seemed appreciative of the fact that clergy were taking mental health care more seriously.

Being at Elgin State gave me a vivid picture of mental health facilities of that time. I was glad I wasn't going into mental health, but throughout my whole ministry I was greatly indebted to the mental health field and my experience at Elgin State Hospital.

Next Granger traveled to Massachusetts General Hospital where Cabot and Dicks had worked together. (Cabot, 1868–1939, was no longer living.) Granger participated in the first summer school of the new Institute of Pastoral Care.

Rollin Fairbanks, the executive director of the institute, organized the program. Fairbanks, who was to serve as the executive director of the Institute from 1944 until 1950, was a graduate of the Episcopal Theological Seminary in Cambridge. He received clinical training at Worcester State and Massachusetts General Hospital. Fairbanks introduced "the controlled interview," (a form of role playing) to pastoral education. He also developed "dual calling" in which the supervisor accompanied students in making pastoral visits in a general hospital.[6]

Granger:

During the first week at Massachusetts General, the seven other clergy students and I served as orderlies, assisting in bathing and caring for the physical needs of the patients. This helped us get a feel for what was going on inside the hospital. During the last five weeks, we spent the morning seeing patients as student chaplains. During the evenings we wrote up our encounters in a verbatim format.

Every afternoon we met in a small group, which was led by a psychiatrist. We read and then reflected aloud on our cases and on what we had said and done. What an eye opener! It was like a boot camp. I learned things about myself that I hadn't learned before because they talked turkey to us. I wasn't used to people talking back to me and telling me that I didn't do things right. They'd say things like, "Did you notice that you didn't listen to the patient?"

Granger was excited about what he was learning. He was eager to begin his work at Augustana Hospital so he could practice new strategies in his personal work with patients and their families. He also was paying close attention to educational strategies, such as the controlled interview and dual calling. He wanted to create opportunities for parish pastors and seminarians to learn the skills that he saw as essential to providing effective pastoral care, both in the parish and in the hospital.

Getting Started ... Early As Usual

In September 1944 Granger began working at Augustana Hospital. This was before his official starting time, but, as usual, he couldn't wait to get going. At first he commuted from the family's temporary home on the south side of Chicago. Then he and Helen found a duplex in Lincolnwood, a rapidly developing northern suburb of Chicago.

In October, the Rev. John Evans reported in *The Chicago Tribune*, that instead of trying to see all the patients every day, Westberg focused on patients who nurses and physicians felt most needed pastoral care. Evans said Westberg would soon be teaching a course for nurses on the religious aspects of patient care, and there would be intensive courses for active pastors as well as classes for theological students. Further, a new chapel would be built.[7]

On October 29, 1944 Dr. P. O. Bersell, president of the Augustana Lutheran Synod and the National Lutheran Council, presided over

Granger's installation as chaplain of Augustana Hospital. The fact that Dr. Bersell presided over the ceremony meant that the synod was taking Granger's new position seriously. Bersell spoke of the chaplaincy at Augustana as "a unique church mission." This was thought to be the first pastoral installation in which a young, rather than an elderly, Lutheran clergyman was inducted as chaplain.[8]

In the 1940s, the hospital superintendent had a great deal of power, so if you were an innovator, having the superintendent on your side was key. Granger: "The administrator of the Augustana Hospital, E. I. Erickson, was a very tall, quiet man who was like a big brother to me. He encouraged me to do anything I'd like to do in terms of changing the chaplaincy program." Indeed, Granger did just that.

Granger approached patient care as a team effort, rather than as something that chaplains, nurses, and doctors did in isolation from one another: "I frequently made calls on patients with nurses, and we learned from each other. A nurse often accompanied me as I took communion to patients. We were a team," exclaimed Granger.

In the 1940s obedience to authority was emphasized in nursing education (indeed in most teaching).[9] Granger felt it was healthy to question authority and was upset that student nurses and even professional nurses were treated in what he, but not many others, regarded as demeaning ways. Granger:

> When physicians approached the nurses' station on a hospital floor, the nurses would stand at attention. If too many people were trying to get on an elevator in the hospital, nurses would defer to physicians. This really bothered me. Later when nurses started talking about getting baccalaureate degrees, I thought that would be one of the most important advances in nursing because it would enable nurses to work more on par both with doctors and patients. However, many doctors said it was unnecessary for nurses to get baccalaureate degrees, that if they did so their studies would take them away from their work.

These doctors were really uneasy about the prospect of nurses becoming more knowledgeable and competent.

Granger advocated working as a team with physicians, but that was more challenging than partnering with nurses. Physicians weren't accustomed to having clergy on their team, and most were skeptical about what a clergy person could contribute. As he had done when he substituted for Chaplain Christianson, Granger sat with the doctors in the dining hall. He told them the story of why he was serving as a chaplain, but they didn't ask many deep questions and, with rare exceptions, they didn't invite him to join them on rounds.

Granger said, "The nurses knew which patients could use my help. But, for the most part, the doctor would only refer dying patients to me." He had expected to find common ground with Christian doctors, but he noted, "Jewish doctors were actually the most open and ready to work together."

Later Granger met Walter Alvarez, a physician who for many years was editor-in-chief of the journal *Medical Care* and a senior consultant to the Mayo Clinic. Alvarez was not affiliated with Augustana Hospital but had an office nearby. He and Granger became intrigued with each other's work. Granger: "After I got Alvarez to speak to the medical staff at Augustana, some Augustana physicians seemed to be a little more open to listening to my ideas." Over the years, Alvarez mentioned Granger in his syndicated newspaper column titled "Medical Round-up." In one article, Alvarez wrote,[10] "As one would expect, Professor Westberg is a fine man—a friendly man and a delightful person to know. He is a man whom people immediately like and trust and talk to, and from whom they get great help. We need many more chaplains like him."

A Persistent Question About Grief

One issue that Granger felt should be of particular concern to chaplains and the health team was grief. In the summer of 1944, when

Granger studied at Massachusetts General Hospital, he had been intrigued with Harvard psychiatrist Erich Lindemann's reflections on the grief experienced by people who had been touched by the devastating Boston Coconut Grove fire of 1942, in which 492 people perished.[11] Granger: "After hearing Lindemann describe what he saw as stages of grief and "grief work," I became attuned to grief, and I saw it all over the place. One of the first things I noted as a hospital chaplain at Augustana was that a lot of the patients were telling me about something they had lost in the past six months or two years—something that was very important to them. And they were grieving about it, although they weren't using the word *grief*. If they had lost a loved one, they would use that word. But they had no idea they could grieve over a smaller loss."

Years later, in writing about his experience at Augustana Hospital,[12] Granger described three patients whom he had cared for and the losses they had experienced before coming to the hospital. Each of these three patients was in the hospital with a "valid scientific diagnosis" of some physical illness. And each one was being treated for the physical symptoms present. None of them was being treated for the grief experiences that may have brought on or exacerbated those symptoms.

As Granger studied the notes he had taken on hundreds of patients, he realized that the illnesses of perhaps one out of every three patients seemed to be related to some significant loss they had experienced in the fairly recent past. Some had lost loved ones. Many had not lost anyone through death, but they had lost something important in their lives, such as a job. Could it be, asked Granger, that this latter group was experiencing deep grief, much like a person who has lost a loved one? Granger:

> Was there a close resemblance between the grief syndrome related to death and the grief related to any significant loss? Little by little I realized that I was spending a large part of my

ministry in the hospital as a grief counselor. Indeed, the grief syndrome always included physical symptoms.

After a year or two I got up sufficient courage to ask the medical staff for an opportunity to present a paper at one of their regular scientific staff meetings. After some months, they granted me a ten-minute spot. In that brief time I tried to convey my hunch that perhaps a third of the patients I was seeing were there in close relationship to some loss they had experienced. I suggested that many of the patients really needed grief counseling. The doctors were not impressed by my insights.

Granger was disappointed, but he recalled, "I kept asking the question." Several years later while raising the issue yet again with a group of nurses at another hospital, Granger got a positive response. "The nursing staff created a questionnaire that they gave to 300 patients. This questionnaire included questions about loss—things that might have happened in these people's lives in the past two years or so. They found that 38 percent of the patients were immediately able to identify some experience that was so traumatic that it caused a life change which had quite possibly made them vulnerable to illness."

Granger was intrigued and continued to think about the possible link between grief and illness. This led to his thinking more intentionally about promoting health before a crisis occurred and educating people about ways to respond to life's inevitable challenges in healthy ways. Granger wanted Augustana Hospital not only to care for sick people but also to foster health and prevent illness by serving as a resource to lay people and clergy in the community.

Community Outreach

As part of hospital community outreach, which was not common in those days, Granger set up a three-hour class for engaged couples, focusing on the "physical, religious, and emotional factors in a marriage," including sexuality.[13] The class, which Granger co-taught with a physician, was intended to supplement the local ministers' premarital counseling sessions.

Granger also had classes for local parish pastors. Granger: "Most ministers agreed that it was important to counsel with couples before they married, but many expressed a need for help with this, especially with the conversations about sexuality. Sexual issues were not openly or widely discussed in that era, even in seminaries. I, as a pastor who had also been in the position of trying to counsel couples, was very sympathetic with the pastors' concerns."

Clergy who valued the class for pastors urged Granger to develop a list of questions on a broad range of topics (not just sexuality) that pastors could use in guiding their discussions with couples. The list of questions that Granger developed was so successful that he was asked to have it published so that it could be more widely available. In 1949 the "Guide" was printed in *The Lutheran Companion*.[14]

Granger then wrote a booklet for ministers that included not only questions for couples but also discourses on the need for premarital counseling, ways of conducting premarital counseling, content for the minister's conversations with couples, and counseling the newly married. The booklet titled *Premarital Counseling* was published in 1950. Eight years later, the National Council of Churches asked Granger to update the booklet, which they then published. Granger also wrote a booklet, titled *Mixed Marriage*, which focused primarily on marriages between Protestants and Roman Catholics.

Granger: "For decades after the booklets were published, whenever I spoke at national meetings, pastors came up to me and told me how they were using the booklets in counseling couples."

In addition to equipping clergy, Granger felt nurses had a great deal to offer and that providing them with additional education would expand the contribution they could make to health teams. He wrote:[15] "There is much more to her work than the technical aspects of caring for the bodily needs of her patients. She spends much more time with the patient than either the physician or the pastor, and she is often in the room at the very moment when the patient is wrestling with inner spiritual problems."

Given the nurses' important roles, Granger developed a course in religion and health for the nursing students who were part of the nursing school established in 1894 and linked to Augustana Hospital.[16] Soon the course was required in each year of the three-year nursing program, making it perhaps the first nursing school in the country to have this kind of requirement.

Some of the topics Granger and his students addressed included the needs of the whole person, the use of prayer and sacraments in the sick room, the parish pastor in the hospital, and the chaplain-nurse team. About teaching nurses, Granger said: "I asked the nursing students to write about the stories of their encounters with patients, using Russell Dicks's verbatim case write-up method of teaching faith-centered counseling. In addition to writing down the conversation, I asked them to indicate what people were doing with their bodies and voices. The nurses were intrigued with this patient-oriented approach."

Years later Granger wrote a book titled *Nurse, Pastor, and Patient*[17] in which he devoted chapters to these and other topics. The book was used as a text not only at Augustana Hospital but also in many other nursing education programs in the United States, Sweden, and other countries.

Advocating Real World Education for Clergy

As Granger traveled around the country giving talks to theological students, clergy, and others, he spoke about his conviction that clergy should have clinical education experiences in the hospital. In his enthusiasm, he invited students and clergy to visit him at Augustana Hospital. Many took him up on his offer. In fact, in May 1945, Granger wrote a letter to Seward Hiltner who was still executive secretary of the Commission on Religion and Health of the Federal Council of Churches. Granger told Seward that he had been so inundated with visitors that it was interfering with his work. To solve the problem, he had created an intensive one-week course. Already there were more than 20 applications for the eight positions in this first course.

Granger also told Seward that after being on the job seven months, he finally had had a chance to address the medical staff of the hospital. "They were very gracious. Since the meeting, referrals from them have tripled. I was careful in my talk to use no terminology that might sound as if I was trying to invade their field or the field of the psychiatrist, and I tried to be as darn humble as I possibly could."

Chapter 7

Whet the Appetite

Granger and Russell Dicks decided to work together on developing curricula for the teaching and learning of clinical pastoral care: Dicks for his already established program; Granger for his new program. Initially Granger focused on ordained ministers rather than seminarians.

Granger conducted his first seminar on pastoral counseling the week of June 18–25, 1945, less than a year after he became chaplain at Augustana Hospital. The course announcement said that the students would focus both on pastoral methods used in hospitals and in counseling people in the parish setting. Granger later wrote:[1] "The goal was to whet the appetite of these clergy to explore the field more carefully in their future work in the years to come."

Every morning the students observed surgery and were given a running commentary by the surgeon. Later in the day there was a classroom lecture by a physician, a nurse, or people such as Russell Dicks and E. I. Erikson, the administrator of Augustana Hospital and president of the American Protestant Hospital Association. Students also made daily pastoral calls on hospital patients. They used the verbatim method to write up their encounters with patients.

During class the students role-played interviews with patients. After the role-plays, Granger and the students reviewed recordings of the interviews that had been captured on a "wire recorder."

In reflecting on the first seminar Granger—predictably—was already thinking about ways to expand the program:[2] "From our experience in this first seminar, it is obvious that such seminars could very easily be conducted in any of the larger church hospitals throughout the country. It is our hope that eventually each of our hospitals will have a chaplain who will consider that a given part of the work ought to be devoted to this type of clinical training."

Even before the first seminar was completed other clergy were clamoring for more courses, so Granger set up three different kinds of courses in "pastoral counseling and ministry to the sick": a five-day seminar for $2.00; a six-week course for $10.00; and a three-month course for fees determined on an individual basis. The courses were open to theological students, parish pastors, and chaplains. Granger: "From the start we took clergy from all denominations, including Roman Catholics. I usually took eight clergy at a time. Most of them had gone through seminary when this kind of clinical education was not available."

Granger explained: "The courses included lectures by doctors on the staff. We wanted students to get a feel for how doctors looked at life, how they treated patients who were dying. Mostly the doctors talked about their particular interests or specialties. Almost all of the lectures ended up in valuable discussions."

A *Chicago Daily News* reporter, Helen Fleming,[3] observed a class in which 15 clergy from eight denominations spent six weeks at the hospital. She quoted Granger as saying, "The minister's biggest fault in personal counseling is that he talks too much. The pastor should let the troubled individual do 75 percent of the talking, but he doesn't. He's so used to preaching that he immediately grabs the conversation by the neck, tells how he handled the same problem in his own life or what the Bible teaches on the subject."

In part, the interest that Granger and Dicks were finding in their courses might have been due to the 8,896 chaplains (2,278 Catholic,

243 Jewish and 5,620 Protestant)[4] who served in World War II and found that their main work was counseling, a task for which they were largely unprepared. In 1944 the Army Chaplain's School, then located at Harvard University, established a curriculum in pastoral care in recognition of this need. When the war was over and the chaplains returned to their parishes and synagogues, many continued to seek help with counseling skills, partially because members of their congregations, influenced by the rising interest in "pop" psychology, wanted this kind of help. By the 1950s, over 80 percent of the Protestant seminaries would offer courses in psychology; some seminaries had at least one psychologist on their faculty.[5]

In 1946, E. I. Erikson, the administrator of Augustana Hospital, and president of the American Protestant Hospital Association (APHA) invited Granger to join him at the annual meeting of the APHA in Philadelphia. This invitation gave Granger the opportunity to work at a national level with Russell Dicks and other colleagues on hospital chaplaincy issues. Several chaplains (Russell Dicks, Albert Hahn, Rollin Fairbanks, John M. Billinsky, and James H. Burns) decided it was time to create a chaplains organization. They proposed that the APHA's constitution and bylaws be amended to provide for a chaplains section. The amendment was adopted at the 1946 meeting.

At the September 1946 APHA Annual Meeting in Philadelphia, Granger joined Dicks and about a dozen chaplains at an organizational meeting during which they adopted their own constitution and named themselves the "Association of Protestant Hospital Chaplains." Dicks was elected president; Granger was elected "chaplain."[6] One of the concerns addressed at that meeting was "consideration of what Protestant hospitals may do to foster cooperation between physicians and ministers." Another was the dearth of good devotional literature for use in the hospitals.[7]

The following year, at the second annual meeting, the Association of Protestant Hospital Chaplains elected Granger as their president.

In 1949 the chaplains association began updating the standards for chaplains, which had been created in 1940 by a commission headed by Dicks. They decided that chaplains should have college and seminary degrees (or the equivalent), ordination, endorsement by their denomination, a minimum of 24 weeks of clinical pastoral education, training in a general or mental hospital, and three years of parish experience or its equivalent.

A Significant Loss

Granger had greatly enjoyed being in close proximity to Dicks, but in 1948 a traditional administrator at Dicks's hospital forced Dicks to move on. Decades later Granger said:[8]

> Russell was on the way to making this prestigious teaching and research hospital [Wesley Memorial] a great Midwest center for what we know now as clinical pastoral education. Then suddenly the administrator[9] who had brought Russell to Chicago died of a heart attack.
>
> Some months later, the new administrator called Russell into his office and asked, "How many patients do you see a day?" Russell countered with, "The question you should ask is, 'How well am I integrating my ministry with the work of the doctors and nurses?'"
>
> But that was not the question. When Russell finally guessed that the number of patients seen by him per day was 10 to 20, the administrator was stunned. "We have 500 patients, and you see only 10 to 20? I think you should see half the patients every day."
>
> The administrator was so serious about this that was the end of Russell's remarkable ministry to Chicago. Many times since those days, I've wondered what would have happened if Russell could have spent the next 35 years developing his action-research style of collaborative ministry with doctors and nurses.[10]

Ahead of His Time

In his first months as chaplain, Granger was way ahead of his time in conceptualizing the work of full-time chaplains as including not only the teaching of nurses, theological students, and clergy but also the teaching of medical students and physicians. In his February 1945 letter to O. V. Anderson, Granger said he thought that the chaplaincy department should provide instruction for medical students and interns in "the art of counseling and the relationship of religion to health."

Granger wrote that medical interns in the average hospital had little or no contact with the religious aspects of illness:[11]

> Seldom are courses taught in their medical schools on this important subject. We feel that the chaplain can at this point in the medical doctor's training make a contribution, which will always be helpful to them. In a formal course of from four to eight hours, he can present case material and histories in which the religious factor has played an important role in the illness. He can point out the correlation between psychotherapy and religious therapy and make clear the role of the Church as an agent in developing a well-integrated individual.

While at Augustana Hospital Granger did not have many opportunities to teach medical students or physicians, but in time he was to do that kind of teaching and exert an impact on a nationally prominent stage.

Creating a Healing Environment

Granger felt that worship and music could be key in helping hospitals be places for healing. Every morning at 6:30 the student nurses at Augustana Hospital were expected to be at chapel, but Granger complained that the main purpose of the service was to make sure that the student nurses' white uniforms were clean and starched, that their hats were in place, and that their white shoes were clean.

A nurse, who some of the students referred to as "the battle ax," stood at the door checking on them. The students were given a little sermonette but little else.

Granger changed the time of the weekday services to noon and invited patients to attend.[12] He told the congregation that they were probably more attentive than most congregations because "this enforced vacation from the frantic pace on the outside has given you the unusual experience of more time to think about those things of spiritual value in your life ... As your chaplain I would be more than happy to help you wrestle with some of the issues you are facing."

Granger also told the congregation that a hospital chapel service provides an opportunity to worship with people from many different denominations. He said that this could happen naturally in a house of healing, a place dedicated to helping all people back to health, no matter what their creed or class or race.

In 1947 Granger was able to bring music into the hospital for weekend chapel services. Viola, Granger's eldest sister, and her family moved to the north side of Chicago, where her husband became pastor of Albany Park Lutheran Church. Granger invited Viola's 14-year-old son to play the organ at the little chapel. John was a gifted musician who played his first wedding on an organ at age nine. Patients and staff were drawn by John's ability to improvise and to inspire people to sing.

Soon there wasn't room for everyone who wanted to attend the chapel service. A new wing was being built for the expanding hospital. Granger proposed that a chapel be built in that wing. E. I. Erickson liked the idea and got the board to agree. Granger was asked to choose the architect and consultants and to help design the chapel.

On December 14, 1948, the cornerstone was laid. The beautiful new chapel, with colorful stained glass windows, seated 150 people. The balcony was designed so that people in wheel chairs could easily see and hear everything that occurred. A small side chapel was open day and night.

Lively Life Lessons

When Granger became a chaplain, he had a long commute to work. Frequently, he had obligations in the evenings and on the weekends. Helen, who was without a car, cared for the house and the family. At a Parent Teacher Association meeting, Granger said some things that Helen undoubtedly wished could occur more in their household.[13] "Mothers of small children ought to get out of the house and away from their children more than they usually do. And fathers of small children ought to get into the house far more than they do."

When Granger was at home, he was a "hands-on" father, playing catch with Jane and John, teaching them to swing a bat, and urging them to polish the car until they could see their faces in it. He also taught them how to empty a mousetrap and pick up snakes. In addition, he shared his love of music. He gave them their first piano lessons. (Some lessons were more successful than others.) While music was playing on the record player, he would pretend to conduct and invite the children to join him in waving their hands to mark the beat. The family always said grace at meals and sometimes had brief devotions afterward. At night, when he was home, Granger would tuck the children in, sometimes telling "Daddy stories"—accounts of when he was a little boy. Sitting on their beds, Granger said evening prayers with the children and occasionally sang with them before he said "Good night."

Much to Helen's relief, sometimes when Granger went into the hospital on weekends, he took one or both of the children with him. John helped clean the chapel. On Sundays he often served as an acolyte. Jane helped Granger's secretary with little jobs. During the car ride Granger would try to engage the children in "serious conversations, listening respectfully to their ideas."

Granger was often asked to give talks about parenting to church groups and parent-teacher groups. Helen told Granger that he should not tell other people how to parent when they were having trouble raising their own children. Apparently, her message got through to him, because he opened one presentation at a PTA meeting by saying:[14] "Now that my children are six and three, I am less able to discuss child psychology. This will be more of a sharing of problems. We always feel better to know that others are having the same difficulties we are."

To illustrate his point, Granger told the following story:

One day I was guest preaching in a large church. Jane and John were sitting up in one of the front rows by themselves. At first they were behaving themselves, but during my sermon, they began getting restless. John started collecting bulletins from the back of the pew in their row. Then Jane joined him in doing this. Pretty soon John crawled under the bench in front of him and got the bulletins there. Then John and Jane both got the bulletins from the row behind them. I could see that John and Jane were getting ready to go across the aisles to get more bulletins. Seeing that they were distracting people, I tried, unsuccessfully, to get them to look at me. Finally, as John was again heading across the aisle, I pointed my finger directly at him, and in a deep voice said, "And the Lord said ..." It worked. John and Jane stopped. But it caused a little snicker in the audience.

After the service, when I saw Jane and John, I said, "Go ahead of me to the car, so it doesn't look like we're together. When you get in the car, duck down in the back seat so that no one will see you."

After Jane and John were out of sight, a deacon came up to me and said, "I want to apologize for those children who disturbed you during the sermon. We don't know who they are but I can assure you it won't happen again."

Every year the Westberg family looked forward to spending one or two weeks at the Augustana Lutheran church camp at Lake Geneva, Wisconsin. Granger had greatly enjoyed camp when he was a boy and wanted his children to have the experience. Young ministers, such as Granger, led the sessions. John and Jane also had some private time with Granger, which he used to teach them to swim, dive, and row a boat. In 1948 Joan Kathleen was born. In time she joined in these activities.

Active Listening

In 1950 Granger was pleased when Seward Hiltner joined the Federated Theological Faculty at the University of Chicago as chair of the department of religion and personality. Granger felt this meant that the University of Chicago was taking the field seriously and that some exciting things would be happening on the campus.

That same year Hiltner invited Granger to join him and others in teaching a course in clinical pastoral education at the University of Chicago under the auspices of the Council for Clinical Training for Theological Students.[15] Granger, as usual, was impressed with Hiltner's abilities: "Seward was one of the brightest men I've ever met. At the end of a daylong seminar or course in which there had been many presentations and much discussion, he could get up and, even without having taken any notes, he could beautifully summarize what had been said. He had a wonderful ability to pull things together."

Hiltner had become one of the most influential leaders in the new field of pastoral care. His book, *Pastoral Counseling*,[16] was widely used in pastoral care courses in North American seminaries. When Seward Hiltner was featured as "the man of the month" in *Pastoral Psychology* in 1951, his 18-year contribution to the field of pastoral psychology was described this way:[17] "There is no man working in the ministry today who has contributed more significantly—both more widely and deeply—to the development, interpretation and application of pastoral psychology in this country."

In 1945, the highly regarded psychologist Carl Rogers joined the faculty of the University of Chicago as professor of psychology. His client-centered approach to counseling and his emphasis on such things as empathy and unconditional positive regard for clients influenced Granger, Seward Hiltner, and many of the leaders in clinical pastoral education. Granger:

> Carl Rogers had planned to go into the ministry. He attended Union Seminary in New York City for a while, but he was disenchanted by the constant discussions about the value of preaching and the lack of attention to counseling. He then went across the street to Columbia University and went into psychology.
>
> Carl effectively demonstrated that clergy tend to preach at people, rather than listen to them. This kind of preaching, of course, turns people off. Carl listened as few people are able to do. He was able to show that active listening coupled with understanding brought about the most helpful results. Learning these things was a major turning point for me.
>
> I attended a course that Carl gave at his home. Most of the other 10 people were psychologists. Carl was a very effective teacher. His teaching method was as important as the content of his teaching. I was very smitten with his approach. He'd give us a little patient case that ended with a statement or question from the patient. Then he'd give us a few minutes to write down how we would respond if we were talking with the patient. When we were finished writing, he would ask us to exchange papers with each other and then, one by one read the answers aloud. (Our names weren't on the papers.)
>
> Ninety percent of the time we would preach at the patient. We got so we'd laugh our heads off because we were doing the absolute wrong things. This was probably one of the most effective teaching methods I'd ever seen because it was done in good spirit, and our responses were anonymous.
>
> Later, I found myself using this method in all my workshops with clergy, even with groups of 100 people. I called it a "What

would you say?" quiz. At first the clergy felt that they had to say the right words so they'd feel like ministers. Finally we'd get to the point where we'd be laughing at ourselves. Even before a response was read, the group would know what was coming. I'd say, "What do you think he said?" and the group would yell out. "Tell him to read the Bible."

Carl's lectures were attended by many theological students who showed more interest in his work and ideas than did the graduate students in psychology.[18, 19] Carl was embarrassed by the attention he was getting from clergy who hung on his every word in the area of personal counseling.

While persisting in learning himself, Granger continued to offer clinical education for pastors. In 1951 Augustana Hospital became affiliated with the Institute for Pastoral Care. The courses at Augustana met all the clinical training requirements of the Institute, so Augustana was one of the sites that the Institute recommended to pastors who wanted clinical training.

In 1952, life changed once again for Granger and his family. Granger: "Out of the blue after being at Augustana Hospital for eight years, I got a phone call from Lowell Coggeshall, dean of the medical school at the University of Chicago. He said, "I heard you speak at a medical meeting the other day, and I was impressed with the new ways you're looking at the chaplaincy program. I'm not very religious, nor is my wife, but we both feel that scientific medicine is so damn cold that we need to warm it up."

Chapter 8

Walls Built So High

In 1952 Granger became the first full-time chaplain of the University of Chicago Clinics.[1] He was also given a faculty appointment: associate professor of pastoral care in the Federated Theological Faculty.[2] This double appointment gave Granger one base in the medical center and another in the schools of theology. The "Clinics," which were administered by the medical school, included outpatient facilities as well as several research hospitals.[3]

After Granger's appointment, the following statement appeared in the *Journal of Medical Education* (the journal of the Association of American Medical Colleges):[4]

Recently, at the University of Chicago Medical School, an interesting experiment has been started. An understanding and experienced young chaplain has been made a member of the staff. He will visit the sick ... and will work with the doctors studying the patients and going over their social and spiritual problems. All deans of medical schools will be interested in seeing how well this experiment works out. It is a fine move forward. A few physicians may be skeptical at first, but in time they probably will be won over.

In an article,[5] Granger outlined five of the duties of the chaplain of a modern hospital. This was, in a sense, his own job description at the University of Chicago.

1. **Ministry to patients.** The chaplain's first concern is the patient. He has learned from experience that he cannot see every patient in the hospital so he must choose those for whom he can do the most good. Doctors and nurses can help him find such people.

2. **Ministry to nurses.** If the hospital has a school of nursing, the chaplain teaches such courses as "The Relation of Religion to Life" and "The Religious Needs of Patients." He also counsels with student nurses who would like to discuss religious and personal problems.

3. **Teaching theological students.** Many hospitals with chaplaincy departments are now opening their doors to theological interns. These young pastors either live in the hospital or come in daily and serve directly under the supervision of the resident chaplain.

4. **Interprofessional relationship.** The hope is that soon there will be regular seminars for physicians and clergymen in which case studies will be presented, which have both religious and physical implications. This approach will help make it clear to the doctor that he must take into account certain underlying religious needs of the patient, and to the clergyman that the physical needs of the patient often color his religious attitudes.

5. **Service to the community.** This includes occasional seminars on "Ministry to the Sick" conducted in the hospital for ministers in the community.

Other community services, Granger wrote, include preaching in local churches and conducting discussion groups on the topic of religion and health for lay people in a variety of settings.

At the University of Chicago Granger was hoping to have more meaningful interactions between clergy and physicians than he had been able to achieve at Augustana Hospital. He was particularly encouraged because Lowell Coggeshall, dean of the medical school, proved to be a strong ally, introducing Granger to key people and taking other steps to support Granger.

Granger knew it would take time to get acquainted with the busy full-time medical faculty of around 200 doctors involved in teaching and research as well as in clinical patient care, but he was optimistic because some physicians invited him to make rounds with them and even included him in the discussions that followed in the classroom. "Being with the doctors in this way gave me the opportunity to discuss the spiritual dimension of patient care," Granger remembered.

Granger was also hopeful that chaplains and physicians in hospitals all over the country would collaborate in the care of people:[6]

> During the past five years more hospitals have placed chaplains on their staffs than during the previous 50 years. Why all this concern for religion in hospitals? ... First there is a growing interest in treating patients in their totality because we are convinced that no patient is "just a body." Second, a growing number of physicians all over the country are asking how religion can give their patients those spiritual strengths which the doctor recognizes to be so necessary in any health or growth process.

Granger's appointment in pastoral care made him one of a growing number of educators in this new field. In 1950, 13 major Protestant seminaries had instructors in pastoral care, including Russell Dicks at Duke, Philip Guiles and John Billinsky at Andover Newton, and Carroll Wise at Garrett Biblical Institute. Writing in a medical journal, Granger described "pastoral care" in this way:[7]

> In addition to preaching to large groups of people from his pulpit, the minister is realizing the importance of ministering to his parishioners individually, as does the doctor. This relationship with people is called pastoral care, and it stresses the minister's role as "shepherd."

Clinical Education for Theological Students and Pastors

Not too long after Granger came to the university, he began to provide real world clinical education opportunities in the clinics and hospitals for theological students and pastors. He expanded the chaplaincy services by having divinity students care for patients, under the supervision of faculty from the theological and the medical schools. Most of the students were full-time theological students taking a yearlong course titled, "Clinical Approach to Pastoral Care." This course marked the first time that students from the theological schools on the University of Chicago campus had formal clinical experiences in the university hospital. Seward Hiltner, of the Federal Council of Churches in America, described the course as "the first instance of such close cooperation between a medical school and a theological school within the same university."[8]

The yearlong course began with a brief stint of orderly work, emptying bedpans, lifting and transporting patients, cleaning, and more. Then, from time to time, the students observed surgery, attended autopsies, and sat in on medical conferences.[9] Every day the student chaplains saw their patients and wrote up their cases, verbatim style. Then in class they presented and discussed their patient cases with Granger and their classmates. Occasionally faculty from the theological or medical school—or both—joined the class.

Each student was attached to a particular doctor's service and was part of a team, which usually included one or two medical residents, two or three interns, and five or six medical students. The team took care of about 20 patients. Physicians invited student chaplains to join their weekly rounds on patients. Granger wrote that physicians did this in part to remind physicians of the availability of chaplains. This practice also reminded the young clergy that physicians are interested in whole patients but find it humanly impossible to minister to every facet of patients' needs.[10]

Although Granger wrote and spoke most often to Protestant audiences, he was also interested in what Jews and Roman Catholics were doing in religion and health, and he spoke to audiences of lay people and clergy from these faiths.[11] His ecumenism is reflected in an article he wrote for the journal of the Central Conference of American Rabbis.[12] Granger acknowledged that some rabbis hesitated to make hospital calls and suggested a number of reasons why they might want to consider making this a regular part of their ministry:

> As ministers of religion, our very presence in the sick room reminds the patient, his relatives, and medical and nursing personnel that religion is concerned about the whole of life ... The rabbi knows that in early Greek communities both religion and medicine were combined in the same person—the priest-physician of the Aesculapian temples.[13]
>
> When a person was being treated by one of these men, he was given both spiritual and physical care. The rabbi wants to make sure that his patient will also receive both kinds of care. He knows that there is always the danger that only the patient's body is being treated because of the present division of medicine and religion.

Granger noted that unlike other professionals, who see people only in times of crisis, rabbis and other clergy are concerned with people from the day they are born until they die. Therefore, they can help members of their congregations put their experiences in perspective, and they can help hospitalized members use their time in the hospital for spiritual exploration and growth.

Challenges of Urban Living

While Granger was adjusting to his new life at the university, he and the family were adjusting to life in the multicultural urban environments in the Woodlawn and Hyde Park communities of the University of Chicago. Before moving from the suburbs, Granger and Helen had prepared 11-year-old Jane, 8-year-old John and 3-year-old Joan for the changes. They emphasized that in their new school and community they would have a chance to meet and make friends with a diverse group of children. However, because of the relatively higher crime rate, Granger and Helen put more restrictions on when and where the children could play in the neighborhood.

A big plus with the move was the fact that Granger didn't have a long commute and could walk to work, giving him more time with the family. Dan Williams was still on the faculty of the Chicago Theological Seminary. He and Granger's sister Lael lived within walking distance, so there was time with extended family.

Early on Granger and Helen invited faculty and students to the house for evenings of conversation. The children were encouraged to greet the company and help serve refreshments, but then they were expected to go to their rooms on the second floor. Granger and Helen were aware that the children sometimes hid quietly on the staircase so they could hear the conversations. Unless it was very late, they let them listen—if they remained quiet.

Granger's parents also lived near the Westbergs' new home. Granger looked forward to visiting them more frequently. However, not long after moving to the University of Chicago, Granger's 87-year-old old father, John, died. Granger: "My father had a very loving attitude and was always upbeat. He could say a great deal in short sentences. He never over-talked. He was a quiet man and a good man. Sometimes he would get a tear in his eye. He never put on airs, even when he took over the company. He never complained, and he was almost never sick."

During the Westberg family's first summer in Woodlawn, tension in the neighborhood was growing. Real estate people were advising neighbors to sell their homes because, they warned, an influx of people from the South was going to bring down the value of their homes. Granger and Helen didn't know it at the time, but these real estate people were deliberately trying to create panic so people would sell their homes for less than they were worth. The homes could then be divided into smaller dwellings and sold to the newcomers on a contract basis that enabled real estate people, bankers, and others to make big profits.[14]

After the summer break, when Jane and John returned to Fiske Elementary School for their second year at Fiske, some of the children from the South, because of previous inadequate schooling, were functioning academically far below the Chicago school system's standards. While teachers worked at bringing these children up to speed, John read library books, and Jane did secretarial work in the principal's office.

The upheaval in the neighborhood was reflected in the school. There were many fights in the classroom and on the playground. John was beaten up at least once. In front of Jane, some new girls threatened Jane's best friend with a switchblade. Granger and Helen met with the teachers and the principal, who told them that they were so busy helping some of the newcomers that they couldn't give John and Jane the attention they needed. They planned to skip them ahead a grade but hoped that Granger and Helen could afford to send them instead to the University of Chicago Laboratory School.

The family budget was tight, but Granger and Helen sent John to the Lab School that next semester. The following September they also started Jane at Lab School. This was the school that John Dewey opened in 1896 to test his new ideas about education. Granger was intrigued by ideas that included experiential learning and encouraging students to ask questions and to be critical thinkers. Many of Granger's colleagues sent their children to Lab School, so there was a sense of community. A few years later Joan started first grade at Lab School.

For Helen, one of the brighter sides of living on the campus was attending the Faculty Wives Club meetings where she was with interesting and stimulating women. However, her travel in the evening to club meetings was not without risk. It was even dangerous to walk from a parking place on the street to the family's house. Helen: "When I was ready to come home, I would call Granger, and he would stand on the front porch and watch as I parked and then walked into the house."

The Westbergs enjoyed having Dan and Lael nearby, but Dan was courted both by Union Theological Seminary in New York City and by Harvard University. In February of 1954, Dan resigned from the Chicago Theological School and accepted the invitation to Union, one of the leading seminaries in the United States.

Yes, More Changes

A bit uneasy about his family's welfare, Granger continued working hard. As a faculty member in the Divinity School, he was on the staff of Rockefeller Memorial Chapel, a beautiful neo-Gothic cathedral, with a world-class organ, choir, and carillons. Located in the heart of the university, weekly worship services and other events were held at the chapel. Granger was impressed with some of the current activities of the chapel, but he felt that with certain enhancements (he proposed a list of 24), the chapel could become even more of a gathering place for the academic and neighborhood communities and that it could draw people from all over Chicago. (Later Granger's son, John, said he didn't know whether Granger handed his list of 24 suggestions to the dean of the chapel or nailed them to the chapel door.)[15]

The dean didn't rush to make all of Granger's suggested changes, but one change was eventually accepted and implemented—namely, the lighting of the chapel at night. In fact, when Nelson Rockefeller visited the campus one evening and saw Rockefeller Memorial Chapel beautifully lit, he requested night lighting of Riverside Church, another cathedral his father, John D. Rockefeller, had built in New York.

When the night lights went on at Riverside Church, Lael and Dan were living in faculty housing at Union Seminary, next door to Riverside Church. Lael was not pleased with having the light shine in their window. She called Granger to tell him she was upset. She ended by saying sarcastically, "I can't imagine whose idea it was to have bright lights on the church at night." For once, Granger was speechless.

Lutheran Connections

In February of 1954, Granger became a member of the editorial advisory board of *Pastoral Psychology*, a journal which, since its establishment in 1950, had featured articles by key figures in psychology, psychiatry, and the social sciences (such as William Menninger, Karen Horney, Erich Fromm) as well as leaders in pastoral counseling. Others on the board included theologian Paul Tillich; Carroll Wise of Garrett Biblical Institute; Russell Dicks at Duke; and Wayne Oates at Southern Baptist Theological Seminary. Carl Rogers was a regular contributor and had been on the editorial advisory board. Seward Hiltner, who played a key role in establishing, shepherding, and writing for the journal, was the pastoral consultant. In later years, when Granger was still on the board, Daniel Day Williams (Granger's brother-in-law) and anthropologist Margaret Mead joined the board.

Granger was listed as a member of the Lutheran Advisory Board and described as "active in almost everything within the Lutheran churches having to do with pastoral care."[6] Although he was on 16 committees at one time, in general, Granger preferred not to be on committees because, as he said, "I enjoy the people on the committees, but usually I prefer doing something rather than just talking."

Granger's Lutheran connections continued. In 1954 Anders Nygren, the esteemed Bishop of Lund, Sweden, was to receive an honorary doctoral degree from the University of Chicago. Nygren, a prominent figure in the Lutheran World Federation and the World Council of

Churches, was being honored for his international ecumenical work.
Granger:

> I had been given the honor of introducing him on behalf of the
> faculty of the Divinity School at the commencement, which
> was held at Rockefeller Chapel. I don't know when I've been as
> nervous as I was at that time as I anticipated this great event.
>
> I first met Nygren outside of the Rockefeller Chapel,
> where the faculty of about 500 people was assembling for the
> procession into the Rockefeller Chapel. He was a very warm,
> personable man, who was easy to talk to. Soon Chancellor
> Kimpton joined us. As we were waiting for the procession to
> start, the chancellor asked, "Granger are you going to present
> the bishop in Swedish?" I answered, "No, I can't speak Swedish,
> but I know a song in Swedish." The bishop asked, "What song
> do you know in Swedish?" I said, "I know the student song
> from Lund University." The song is very joyful, so I started
> singing it. Immediately the bishop joined me. As we entered
> the chapel, we came to the final chorus, which ended, "Hurrah,
> hurrah." The good-natured laughter from the faculty and others
> was tremendous.

Bishop Nygren was in Chicago that summer of 1954 so he could
attend the Second Assembly of the World Council of Churches (WCC)
held at Northwestern University in Evanston, Illinois. The WCC,
which was founded by representatives of 147 denominations largely
from North America and Europe, had met for the first time in 1948 in
Amsterdam. It was born out of a desire for visible unity and peace.

Granger attended the WCC meeting. Later in a sermon at Rockefeller
Chapel titled, "A Next Step in Ecumenicity," Granger reported, "It was
a thrilling experience to observe Christians of so many backgrounds
and types working and worshiping together." Granger spoke of the
spirit of openness that characterized the discussions and "the attitude

of humility evidenced by so many ecclesiastical leaders who saw that their own denominations could be enriched by this interchange of religious experience."[17] He said, "Fifty years ago it was thought that such a meeting would be impossible because the walls separating the denominations had been built up so high that each group in its isolation was satisfied with its own denomination as it was."

Granger said he was glad that some Christians were dissatisfied with their divisions and did something about it. "Yet in this remarkable meeting of Christians we were saddened by the absence of a large segment of Christendom. Our Roman Catholic friends were not there, and we missed them. Their presence could have added tremendously to the discussions ... Because of our common loyalty to Christ, it is a tragedy that we are still separated after 400 years. We tend to accept the rift as if it were meant to be permanent. It is not!"

Granger said that even though the Roman Catholic Church turned down the invitation to go to Evanston, unofficial discussions could take place at all levels, and that these unofficial discussions could "lay the foundation for future official actions."

Uniting Lutherans

Granger was also eager to see walls broken down between the various Lutheran traditions. For many years Granger had been eager for the Lutherans from the Augustana Synod and other synods to join together and have a presence on the University of Chicago campus. He argued that the study of theology should not take place on isolated campuses. Rather, seminary faculty and students should be in an environment where they would be stimulated by the points of view of people from other fields and faith traditions. He wanted Lutheran faculty and students to have the resources of a great university. He also felt that Lutherans had a contribution to make.

In 1953, Granger helped arrange for the seminary to hold the Lutheran ordination service at Rockefeller Memorial Chapel so the faculty members, seminarians, families, and delegates from around the United States could become acquainted with the beautiful chapel and campus. The cathedral-sized chapel was filled, with standing room only for 800 people outside.

The next year Granger arranged for his longtime friend, O. V. Anderson, to be installed as the new president of the Augustana Synod at Rockefeller Chapel. The service again brought many Lutherans to the campus. Unfortunately, afterward, while Anderson and others were celebrating at the Westbergs' home, all of Anderson's new vestments were stolen from his car.

In 1957 Granger led a successful effort to reserve land in the University of Chicago community for the Lutheran School of Theology.[18] Four Lutheran synods were talking about merging three Midwestern synods of Scandinavian ancestry[19] plus the largest synod, the United Lutheran Church in America (ULCA), of German roots. The three synods of Scandinavian background each had one seminary. The ULCA had 10 regional seminaries, including four in the Midwest. In 1958 as the talks on merging the churches progressed, the boards of Augustana Seminary and the Chicago Lutheran Seminary at Maywood (ULCA) created an Inter-Seminary Committee to plan the future of the seminaries. Granger was on the committee. He was pleased that the relatively small Suomi Seminary (Finnish) was already in the process of moving to the Maywood campus. Two years later the small Danish seminary also moved to the Maywood campus. This was a start, but Granger strongly advocated moving these three seminaries and Augustana Seminary to a consolidated seminary on the University of Chicago campus.

After more than a decade of heated discussions and gradual movement, most of the Lutherans did get together on property adjacent the University of Chicago campus. They called themselves the Lutheran School of Theology at Chicago. This didn't happen, though, until 1967, after Granger had left Chicago for new horizons.

Still Thinking About Nurses

Meanwhile, Granger had an unfinished project that was also related to breaking down walls and helping people work together. Even though Granger was no longer working with a school of nursing, he was still pursuing his vision of nurses and clergy working together in the care of patients. He had written some articles[20] but wanted to pull his thinking together in a book.

With his busy life, Granger was not making much progress. He needed a retreat away from his workplace. He and Helen also wanted a summer retreat where their four children (Helen Jill, called Jill, was born in 1954) could play safely and all of them could escape the summer heat of Chicago. In the summer of 1955 Granger and Helen bought a small cabin a mile from Lake Geneva, where they had honeymooned and both had family histories. The cabin was across the lake from Camp Augustana, where they had taken the family for a couple of weeks every summer. Often, they had looked longingly at other people's summer homes. Now they had their own.

To afford the cottage, Granger and Helen rented the first two stories of their Chicago house to graduate students for the summer. On the weekends Granger joined the family at the lake, but during the week, when he was in Chicago, he had to stay in the bedroom on the hot third floor. While Granger was in town Helen did not have a car at the lake and had to call on neighbors when there were unplanned events, such as a rushed trip to the doctor when Joan got hit on the head with a baseball bat during a neighborhood game. Helen had to wash Jill's diapers by hand. All of them had to walk a mile to the lake where they swam once or twice a day. Nevertheless, Granger and Helen felt these challenges were worth it.

On weekends, during that summer at the cottage, Granger finished writing *Nurse, Pastor, and Patient*. He noted that the nurse, as a frontline professional, was closest to patients for the longest period of time and thus was in a unique position to get to know patients and be helpful to them. Patients could temporarily put on "company manners" for others, such as physicians, ministers, priests, rabbis, and relatives who paid brief visits, but during the course of several days, the nurse was likely to know patients in all of their moods. "Intuitively," wrote Granger, "she seems to know how to be at the patient's side at just the right time." This puts her in a unique position to help patients not only with their physical problems but with their psychological problems and with their problems "of the human spirit." Also, because of the nurse's unique position in relation to the patient, physician, and minister, "she is able to sense what a patient needs most and how a minister can be a part of the healing team."

Granger felt that since nurses were in such a key position, they should be educated "in the art of conversation" so as to be "of real help to patients who are going through inner struggles." These skills, he said, "will be just as important in her task as the work that she does with her hands or with her knowledge of pharmacology." With these skills "nursing can take on a dimension that contributes immeasurably to the healing process."

As Granger worked on *Nurse, Pastor, and Patient*,[21] he invited Helen and 14-year-old Jane to read the manuscript and give him feedback. Granger greatly valued Helen's opinions. He also listened respectfully to Jane's ideas.

Nurse, Pastor, and Patient was largely devoted to the topics Granger dealt with in the classes he conducted for nurses at Augustana Hospital. One topic, the needs of the whole person, was not widely discussed at that time. Granger wrote: "The body can never be sick by itself, nor the psyche by itself, because man is one. Spirit means, in fact, the whole person."

Granger also noted that the word *psychosomatic* is not hyphenated. This he said "points up the fact that any approach to illness ought to take into account that a person can never be split up into two parts: with the doctor taking care of the body and minister dealing with the spirit. The two are inseparable."

In his nationally syndicated newspaper column, Dr. Walter C. Alvarez wrote that *Nurse, Pastor, and Patient* was "a splendid little book on the relation between the nurse, the pastor and the patient." He said that it "should be in the hands of every nurse and hospital chaplain. It shows how much difference there is between caring for the sick and caring for them with kindness and a feeling of consecration."

Granger dedicated *Nurse, Pastor, and Patient*,[22] to Helen, "my understanding counselor." Granger: "I had taken on so many things that I would wake up at night feeling very tense. Helen would listen to my concerns. I would then turn over and fall into a deep sleep while she stayed awake. Helen was such an effective counselor that I didn't need to go to a professional. She had an unusual maturity and was filled with good ideas."

Union Seminary?

Granger's sister Lael and her husband, Dan, were still at Union Theological Seminary. Entries in Lael's diary in late 1955 reveal that Union was courting Granger. On December 21, 1955, she wrote that Granger met all day with the faculty. Granger's December 30, 1955 letter to President Van Dusen, however, reveals that although he was intrigued with Union's new program, he turned down the invitation to join the faculty.

> Since returning home I have had talks with four of our key people related to the program in which I am engaged. All of them assure me that the years of building a foundation are now past and that we are ready to go to work on the superstructure. Despite the intriguing possibilities in the Union project, I feel "called" to remain here at the University of Chicago and see this project through. I feel that now I am beginning to belong to the medical as well as the theological faculty.

Some faculty members at Union persisted. On January 6, 1956, the Committee on Psychology and Religion voted to recommend

Granger as full professor at Union. On February 10, Granger again turned down Van Dusen, indicating that he was very tempted by the offer but that the University of Chicago had asked him to take a newly created professorship in religion and health. Later Granger recalled, "This was a somewhat difficult decision to make, but I felt Union could not offer the unique relationship to a medical school that I enjoyed at the University of Chicago."

Granger still had dreams of ministers and doctors working collaboratively in the care of patients. He was making some modest progress. He thought his opportunities to help make that happen were greater at the University of Chicago than at Union Seminary, which wasn't associated with a medical school.

Linked to his dream of ministers and doctors working together was the vision of divinity schools and medical schools working together to prepare students of theology and medicine to work together. Speaking of the University of Chicago campus Granger said, "The divinity school and the medical school were on the same campus, only about 300 feet apart, but they could just as well have been 300 miles apart. There had been no communication between them, ever." Granger was eager to build bridges between the schools.

Chapter 9

A Pioneering Joint Appointment

In June 1956, Granger was given a joint appointment in both the Federated Theological Faculty and the school of medicine at the University of Chicago. One of his explicit and welcomed tasks was to try to build bridges between the two schools. Granger also was given tenure, a sign that the university thought highly of his work and supported him. *Time Magazine* took note of the appointment.[1]

The University of Chicago announced the appointment of the Rev. Granger Westberg to a new post: professor of religion and health. Lutheran Westberg, 42, chaplain for the past three years at the university's clinics and before that at Chicago's Augustana Hospital, will serve on both the medical and theological faculties, putting into practice his conviction that patients' physical, mental and spiritual health are all of a piece, and that medicos and ministers should work together.

An article in *Pastoral Psychology*[2] noted that Lawrence Kimpton, chancellor of the University of Chicago, said this joint professorship in religion and health was believed to be the first of its kind. Dr. Lowell Coggeshall, dean of the school of medicine was quoted as saying, "Under this joint appointment more study can be made of the proper relationship between the physician and the minister as they seek to help people. The Rev. Mr. Westberg's services will be available to help the medical students understand through informal seminars and some formal instruction what the clergy can do for patients."

Jerald C. Brauer, dean of the Federated Theological Faculty, said he considered the appointment to be "a pioneering development in both medical and theological education, for the appointment recognizes that both theology and medicine are concerned with the same person. The patient is a human being whose welfare involves spiritual as well as physical and mental health. With this established means of cooperation, doctors and ministers can learn from each other. By bringing theological and medical students together in their education program, the appointment can have great impact on both professions."

Recognizing his pioneering work, in June 1956, Augustana College gave Granger an honorary doctorate. Although Granger was working in an ecumenical world, the Lutheran church was still his "family," so he felt greatly honored to be acknowledged by his alma mater.

New Colleague

During Granger's initial four years at the university, the chaplaincy department and its educational program had become an established part of hospital life. An increasing number of physicians referred patients to the chaplains. Theology students served as assistant chaplains, working with patients under the supervision of faculty members. Granger was delighted with this progress but needed time to pursue his new responsibilities, so Carl Wennerstrom, a Unitarian minister and a PhD candidate in theology, was appointed chaplain of the University of Chicago Clinics.

In his new role, Granger continued seeing some patients and doing some teaching in the chaplaincy training program, but now he was able to spend more time making rounds with doctors and medical students and creating opportunities for dialogue between the medical school and the Federated Theological Faculty.

Granger's pioneering appointment came right before the summer break, giving him the summer in which to plan the upcoming school year. Carl Wennerstrom was one of the people with whom he strategized. They were able to do this at Lake Geneva. The previous summer Granger and Helen had introduced the Wennerstroms to the joys of the lake. The Wennerstroms bought Granger and Helen's old cabin, and Granger and Helen arranged to have a new cabin built that would better accommodate their family of six. When the cabin was completed, Granger wanted to participate in building a kitchen table and bunk beds. Carl was an excellent carpenter and was able to guide Granger. Even as they worked with their hands, they continued to plan the new school year.

Expanding the Vision

Granger was eager for medical schools beyond the University of Chicago to open their doors to the teaching of religion and medicine. In part because of his new joint appointment, in November of 1956 he had the opportunity to promote this idea when he gave a keynote address to the audience of more than a thousand leaders in medical education from around the world at the 67th annual meeting of the Association of American Medical Colleges (AAMC), the premier organization in medical education in the United States.

Granger:[3]

> During the past 10 or 15 years some rather unexpected things have happened in the relationship between medicine and religion. Ministers and physicians who previously have had only a speaking acquaintance are now discovering that they have quite a bit in common—namely, the patient; and so they are beginning to converse on a professional level.
>
> ... There has been a growing interest in the patient as a person, a whole person, with physical, mental and spiritual needs, which somehow do not respond well to piecemeal

treatment. A great many physicians, seeing the needs of the whole patient, are seeking new ways to minister more effectively to all these needs.

The clergy's role was also changing, Granger said. The minister was comfortable preparing and delivering lectures and sermons, and theological education prepared clergy well for these tasks. But now "his parishioners are demanding that he get down out of his pulpit and work with them and their problems down where they are." This kind of counseling with people was not a task that theological education previously addressed.

Granger described how, in an attempt to prepare seminarians for their new roles, theological schools had been starting to require students to engage in supervised clinical experiences:

It is no secret that theological educators are indebted to medical education for demonstrating how theory may be made relevant to practice, by daily moving back and forth between classroom and clinic. In addition to this, theologians, recognizing that they never minister to a soul apart from a body, have invited physicians to participate in the instruction of theological students.

Now that theological schools profit by the presence of mature physicians in their classrooms and clinics, could it be that medical students might profit from having qualified clergymen related in some way to the educational program?

Granger said later, "When I finished my presentation to the medical educators at the AAMC meeting, they gave me a standing ovation. I thought they were anxious to catch their planes. Then I began receiving invitations to medical schools. For some of them it was the first time they had been confronted with a person who raised and discussed religious issues. Since I would go to a medical school for a day or two, hit them with some ideas, and then leave town, some people called me the hit-and-run professor."

Granger's visits to medical schools were not a short-lived phenomena. Three years later an article in the *AMA News* (American Medical Association News) reported large turnouts of enthusiastic students at the medical schools of the University of Pennsylvania, the University of Rochester, and the University of Iowa for Granger's lectures on religion and health. "We are seeing a renewed and vigorous interest by the medical profession in the interrelationship of medicine and religion in treating the whole patient," the article stated.[4]

Teaching classes for medical students was one way that Granger tried to bridge the gap between religion and health at the University of Chicago medical school. In five required classes for second-year medical students, Granger focused on areas of potential cooperation between ministers and doctors. He also taught an elective course in religion and health, focusing on such topics as the relationship of morals and medical practice; the relationship between faith, grief, and illness; guilt; faith healing; religious views on sexuality and birth control; terminal illness; and the relationship between religion and psychiatry.

Bimonthly religion and medicine case conferences were a strategy Granger used to bring the medical and the divinity schools closer together. Physicians, nurses, social workers, and chaplains, along with individuals in training for those professions, attended these brownbag noon conferences. Granger wrote,[5] "The conferences are clinical in nature, and they center on a particular patient who is being seen by members of these professions. The format of each conference is the discussion of the patient from various perspectives, with special emphasis on the religious dimensions of the patient's life and the way in which the patient's attitudes toward life contribute to his illness and health."

A student chaplain in the one-year course in clinical pastoral care, and the health team with which he was working, selected the case to be featured at each conference. Granger recalled: "The doctor was invited to present the case at the conference in the customary way. The physicians were asked to lead off because they were not accustomed to involving nurses and chaplains in the process. Then the nurse would talk about the patient from her point of view. Finally the student chaplain would make a presentation."

Years later during an interview Granger said,[6] "In the beginning we had to force ourselves to deal with the spiritual dimension of illness. It was difficult. It was much easier to talk about the physical and psychological elements. We had to call ourselves back again and again. We found that we didn't have a religious vocabulary we could use to discuss the spiritual in an interdisciplinary group. Religious concepts such as 'grace' and 'justification by faith' were a part of a foreign language in that setting."

Elsewhere Granger wrote:[7]

Even when we brought in top-flight theologians from the theological faculty of the university, they had difficulty applying religious dimensions to a patient's clinical situation. But we worked at it week after week, and sometimes it became quite an effective means of education. We chaplains felt good about this new interchange between doctors and ministers. Prior to that, we had seen the doctor only in the role of the captain of the team, or as a lecturer to our group where we dutifully took notes. The doctor was clearly in charge. We were not sure where we stood as members of the health team—or if we were really on it!

The conferences provoked a variety of reactions. Granger:

Some doctors left the conferences scratching their heads and saying, "How did they get me involved in this unscientific approach to illness?" But others said, "This is the first time I've ever even thought about the religious dimension of my patients' illnesses. And it's the first time I've sat down on an equal footing with nurses and pastors and had to slug it out with them!" The nurses said, "This is what ought to happen every day on the hospital floors." They kept urging me to expand the concept.

Reflecting on the conferences, Granger noted that nurses served as intermediaries between clergy and physician:[8] "In those case conferences, we pastors and the physicians attempted to learn how to talk with each other. We soon learned that we lived in two different worlds and spoke two quite different languages. It was the nurses who helped in the translation. As we gradually got over the language barrier, with the help of nurse interpreters, our discussions became more valuable."

Granger was disappointed that the religion-medicine case conferences were not moving more quickly in bridging the gap between ministers and doctors, but he did notice some small gains. "At the end of each conference," Granger said, "doctors would frequently say things like, 'It's been interesting to learn what you folks are actually saying and doing for our patients.' But there was no great clamor on their part to include us in the diagnostic workup of their patients. Yet we did notice on the floors a little more willingness to talk to us about certain patients."

Ideas for Theological Education

Granger was exposed to the then current medical education model, in which theory and practice began to be blended at the end of the second year of medical school. Granger argued that theory and practice must also be blended in theological education. He speculated about what the "ideal day in the life of a middler or senior seminarian" would look like if theological education used the medical education model.[9]

In the morning this seminarian would be in the classroom "where basic subjects are taught." In the afternoon, he would be in a clinical situation (medical center, social agency, parish, senior community, children's home) where, under supervision he would "give pastoral care to the living, breathing human beings who are going through moments of crisis." In the evening, the seminarian would be in the library digging out answers to questions that had been raised during the day. Late evenings would find the seminarian engaged with colleagues "in traditional bull sessions where insights gained both from theory and practice would be talked over and integrated into a meaningful pattern." Granger said, "Whenever such a balanced diet of theory and practice is possible, the student finds himself listening more attentively than ever to the morning lectures. He does not sit in class primarily to get academic credit. He is there to get insights because now someone on the outside to whom he is related in a spiritual ministry is depending on him."

International Opportunities

Granger was getting international inquiries and invitations, particularly from people in Sweden and the United Kingdom. Because of his strong family ties to Sweden, Granger was especially interested in getting to know Sweden and using it as a base of operation for future trips. One of his dreams was to make it possible for a Swedish psychiatrist and a Swedish pastor to study for a year at the University of Chicago. With help from Bishop Nygren and others, Granger arranged a trip starting in August 1958.

Granger began his trip in Edinburgh and London where, with some notable exceptions, he found that clergy and physicians were not very open to his new ideas. The first of three medical schools that Granger visited in Sweden was linked to the University of Uppsala, the oldest university of Sweden (founded in 1477). Granger lectured and met with theologians and medical educators. Then he went to the Karolinska Institute in Stockholm, one the most highly regarded medical centers in the world. Granger:

One morning while I was talking with the dean in his office, he said, "We have a professor of internal medicine who is quite opposed to religion. I think you ought to speak to his class." When I agreed, he phoned the professor. As he talked with the professor, I heard the dean say that I was a minister and that I wasn't a fanatic.

When I went up to the professor's room, we had coffee together. He told me that he was a well-known agnostic because for several years he and one of the bishops had been engaged in an ongoing discussion that had been appearing in the newspaper. At the end of our discussion he invited me to speak to his class the next day.

The professor introduced me to his class by saying, "I met this young minister yesterday. I thought you'd like to hear what's going on in America." I had the classes' attention as I spoke about such things as how we're trying to bring physicians and clergy together around the care of the patients. The students' questions showed that they were taking what I said very seriously.

When I finished, the professor said, "We have listened to something that I've never heard of before. And I think Dr. Westberg is a very clever fellow because I can't think of anything I'd disagree with on." I was glad for that. When I present new ideas, I try to speak positively and not antagonize people.

One day Granger had the thrill of visiting the Swedish royal palace and talking with one of the king's men, who listened with interest to Granger's ideas. Later, while standing outside the Swedish parliament building watching Archbishop Hultgren and other church dignitaries process out, he saw Bishop Anders Nygren. In a letter to the family Granger wrote:

When Nygren saw me he dropped out of the procession and gave me a big hug. Then he introduced me to the archbishop and others saying, "This is the man who is speaking at three medical schools in Sweden. I want you to meet him." Nygren had already told Archbishop Hultgren about my work. We spent a good long time talking, and Hultgren asked all the right questions. Believe it or not, he is intensely interested. When he comes to Chicago in 1960, he wants to see some of our programs firsthand.

After getting such a wonderful reception from Archbishop Hultgren, I bumped into Bishop Bo Giertz. As I reported to him what I had been doing, he smiled from time to time and chuckled, then slapped his knee in glee. Finally he put his arm around me and said, "You have done more for the Church of Sweden in three weeks than we could have done in 10 years. We are very, very grateful to you."

Before finishing his professional obligations, Granger went to Karlstad, Sweden, to visit with his cousin Sven Persson and his wife and two sons. Years earlier when Granger and Sven met briefly in the United States, they immediately liked one another. Sven, a bright man who was fluent in eight languages, was a few years younger than Granger. He was an engineer who eventually became president of Scandinavian ESSO. Granger: "Sven, like many Swedes, was not active in a church, but we discussed theology by the hour, and he showed real interest in my work. I think he would have made an excellent minister."

Granger and Sven also reflected about what might have happened if Granger's father had stayed in Sweden and Sven's father had gone to the United States, instead of vice versa. What might Granger have been like if he had been raised in Sweden? What might Sven have been like if he had been raised in the US?

In Lund, Sweden, the birthplace of his maternal grandfather, Granger visited more relatives. At Lund University, he met separately with faculty in the medical school and the department of theology, and he lectured in both schools. The most important outcome of that visit was being introduced to a shy, young theology student, Bertil Werkström, whom the faculty thought had great promise.

Shortly after Granger returned to the University of Chicago, responding to requests from Werkström and his mentors, Granger arranged for Werkström to get a scholarship to the Divinity School. Granger: "Then we got a message that Bertil had gotten married and that his wife, Kerstin, would like to come along and work on her master's degree in nursing. So I got a scholarship for her."

The Werkströms came to the university and studied for one year. Granger and Helen helped them feel at home. As a gift, when the Werkströms returned to Sweden, they translated *Nurse, Pastor, and Patient* into Swedish.[10]

Helen: "The next time that the Werkströms visited us, he was dean in the Church of Sweden. On the visit after that, he was a bishop. Then, on a subsequent visit, he was the Archbishop of the Church of Sweden."

Granger had gone to Sweden to explore the extent to which there was dialogue or collaboration between religion and medicine. Physicians and clergy received him cordially. Many were curious about this clergyman of Scandinavian descent who was teaching in a well-regarded American medical school. They listened with interest to what he said. But as Granger had suspected, most Swedish physicians, like most other Swedish citizens, had little or no contact with the church, and Swedish clergy were doing little or nothing to reach out to physicians or to explore the intersections between religion and health. In part, Granger thought this might be due to that fact that, in many ways, theological education in Sweden was even more removed from real life than in the United States.

Granger enjoyed his time in Sweden, but despite the openness of theological students, medical students, and some of the faculty to his ideas, he did not have great hopes of any exciting collaboration between religion and medicine in Sweden in the near future. Thanks to Bertil and Kerstin Werkström, though, Granger's work with nursing had a legacy in Sweden. He later learned that the Werkströms' translation of *Nurse, Pastor, and Patient* sold well in Sweden and was used in some schools of nursing.

Chapter 10

Working and Learning in Communities

Following World War II, when Granger was chaplain at Augustana Hospital, the public's view of psychiatrists and psychiatry was greatly improved because of the ways in which psychiatrists were able to understand and care for military personnel and veterans. Many state-run "mental hospitals" still existed, but finally more people with mental health problems were being cared for in general hospitals, and psychiatrists were more of a presence in general hospitals. At Augustana, Granger tried to involve a psychiatrist in the clinical education program for seminarians and clergy, but, although he respected the psychiatrist, they could not find an effective way for that psychiatrist to work with the students.

In his early days at the University of Chicago, Granger wrote that he was grateful to psychiatry for its wake-up call. He acknowledged that psychiatrists had taken the lead in caring for people with mental illness and that church hospitals had been slow to accept patients with mental health problems.

In 1957 Granger wrote that while for 2,000 years the church "has concerned itself with broken hearts," it was psychiatry, not the church that was reminding us about this way of thinking.[1]

This experience is good for us ... It is the best jolt we have had in many a year. It hurts our pride to have to admit that men of science have seen some things in the nature of man, which we had overlooked, and that they may have discovered ways to help people back to sanity that we had not found. Harder to accept … is that what these physicians have actually rediscovered is our own basic stock in trade—love—and they have put it at the center of their therapy.

Granger saw the potential in collaboration between psychiatrists and clergy but he was disappointed and even deeply upset sometimes by the way he thought some psychiatrists did not recognize or even debunked the spiritual dimension of health and health care.

Fortunately Granger found a kindred spirit in a few psychiatrists, such as Dr. Edgar Draper, a psychiatrist in the department of psychiatry at the University of Chicago with a master's degree in theology. Draper's focus was the new field of community psychiatry. For decades some people suffering from mental illness were hospitalized for long periods of time, even years. With the advent of psychotropic drugs and better forms of talk therapy, mental health patients were being sent home or to less restrictive settings. Also, mental health professionals were realizing that some illness could be prevented or treated more easily if people at risk for illness, or in the early stages of illness, were identified and supported. This meant some psychiatrists needed to work in the community and see people before they were in more advanced stages of illness.

Granger thought that ministers with appropriate education could potentially be important partners in identifying and caring for people in the community with mental health issues. He pointed out that, typically, psychiatrists did not see people until they were quite ill. In contrast, Catholic, Protestant, and Jewish clergy had firsthand contact with people in all conditions. They saw people at church or at the synagogue and, with the exception of a few physicians, they represented the only profession that regularly made house calls. Draper and other colleagues agreed with Granger that clergy could play an important role. But how could clergy be given the learning experiences needed for recognizing the early stages of mental illness? How could they prepare themselves to work collaboratively with mental health professionals?

The annual two-week long course in pastoral care at the University of Chicago provided some preparation for this work.[2] Headed by Seward Hiltner and taught by Hiltner, Granger and faculty from the theological and medical schools, this course was geared for parish clergy, most of whom had little opportunity during seminary to develop the skills needed for recognizing mental illness and working collaboratively with mental health professionals. Participants typically felt they learned a great deal during the course at the university but thought that implementing what they learned at home could be daunting, particularly because they would not have the support of colleagues who had gone through the same or a similar experience. Speaking for other participants, a pastor from Kokomo, Indiana, wrote in his evaluation of the course, "I wish that every minister in Kokomo could take this course."[3]

Granger knew that a two-week course at a university didn't provide the time or experiences needed for learning the capabilities essential for providing effective pastoral care. Pastors needed multiple opportunities to practice using their new knowledge and skills in their churches and communities, and they needed to share their experiences and reflections and receive feedback from experts and their peers.

Granger was excited by the idea of setting up a program that focused on one community and allowed for follow-through. He, Ed Draper, and their colleagues developed a proposal to bring clergy from all faiths to the university for a week. Then the clergy would go home for six months and "try out" what they learned, meeting regularly as a group to discuss their efforts with their peers and faculty. Following the six months, the pastors would return to the University of Chicago for another week on campus.

Clergy and other professionals in Kokomo, Indiana, as well as faculty at the university, were intrigued with the proposal. Granger and his colleagues secured funding from the Lilly Endowment for what was called the Kokomo Project. Granger's department of religion and health sponsored the project with the assistance of the department of psychiatry. Granger and Chaplain Carl Wennerstrom were directors of the project. Edgar Draper devoted full time to the project during the two weeks that Kokomo clergy were at the university. John Hoyt, a psychiatrist in Kokomo, participated in the entire project.

In June 1958, 24 participants (one Roman Catholic priest and 23 Protestant clergy, representing 10 denominations) spent one week on the University of Chicago campus. (There were no rabbis living in Kokomo at that time.) During each 10-hour day on the campus, ministers attended lectures given by divinity and medical school faculty,[4] engaged in clinical pastoral care in the hospital, read, and wrote up cases. During "whole-group" discussions, participants were challenged with "What would you say?" quizzes. Participants also met in small groups where they role-played minister-parishioner interactions and presented their own cases (either from their parish or from their experiences in the university hospital). The participants (all men) lived together in the same dormitory so could easily get together for conversation.[5,6]

On returning to Kokomo after the first week, the men reported that a new kind of professional relationship developed between them. They expressed a newfound confidence and trust in each other through dependable, personal relationships, a lessening of competition, and a new understanding of the mutuality of their problems. Some said that they were now able to "find a brother confessor to whom I might go with personal problems."

Back in Kokomo, the entire group met monthly for four-hour sessions in which they discussed cases from their congregations with two or three faculty from the University of Chicago and psychiatrist John

Hoyt. After six months of meetings in Kokomo, the group returned to Chicago for a second intensive week on the campus. The group then asked if Granger and his colleagues could continue the monthly clinical sessions in Kokomo, this time devoting two of the four hours in each session to discussions with people from medicine, law, social work and education who worked in Kokomo. Funding was provided, and the project continued with additional positive outcomes. A participant in the Kokomo Project told a *New York Times* reporter, "This experience has helped me feel that we clergymen are partners rather than competitors." The group decided to work together in other ways. For example, they instituted a regular premarital counseling course.[7] Even after the funding for the Kokomo Project was over, the clergy in the project continued to meet on their own to improve their clinical pastoral skills and to support each other.[8]

The model used for the Kokomo Project was also used for the La Grange Project located west of Chicago, where Granger and family had moved in 1959. Granger wrote that the most significant differences between the two projects was that La Grange was home to many executives, and the La Grange pastors were serving "top" churches in their denominations.

In the La Grange Project greater efforts were made to include doctors. At each session, pastors presented cases and received feedback and suggestions from their colleagues. Most of the clergy had never experienced this kind of learning. A few left, but most continued throughout the two years of the project.[9]

Granger wrote that the following were among the goals for both the Kokomo and La Grange Projects:

1. Help clarify the minister's role and responsibility in the search for underlying causes of mental illness.
2. Help prepare parish clergy to recognize emotional problems.
3. Demonstrate the importance of a cooperative focus on mental illness by fellowship and exchange among community pastors.

4. Introduce clergy to other professionals working in the area of health.

5. Encourage pastors to promote an ongoing educational program in their own churches related to mental and spiritual health.

6. Help ministers obtain new insights for their own personal mental health.

In their book, *Community Psychiatry and the Clergyman*,[10] Granger and Ed Draper wrote that although they achieved many of the projects' goals, neither the Kokomo nor the La Grange group continued for the years after the funding period, as they had hoped. In part this was due to the high mobility of clergy, a fact of which they had been unaware when starting the projects. Indeed, a few years after the projects, only a handful of the clergy participants were still living in Kokomo or La Grange.

Meanwhile, Granger was on to other projects. In particular, he wanted to ensure that during seminary, students were effectively prepared to be helpful to people with mental health and other issues.

Proposing Radical Changes

For years, as a faculty member at the University of Chicago and as a member of the boards of Augustana Seminary and the American Association of Theological Seminaries, Granger had been calling for changes in theological education that would better prepare seminarians for the real world. None of the groups he addressed over the years had yet been ready for what he had to say. Some people, in fact, were irritated by his suggestions. The Kokomo and La Grange Projects had made clear that many pastors did not feel they had been sufficiently prepared during seminary for counseling parishioners and other tasks.

In the late 1950s, Hans Hofman, a professor of theology at Harvard University, asked Granger to contribute a chapter to a book he was editing on new directions in the education of ministers.[11] Granger titled his chapter, "The Need for Radical Changes in Theological Education: A Proposed 44-Month Plan."[12] In the foreword to Granger's chapter, Hofman wrote:[13] "The editor wishes to express his full sympathy with Westberg's suggestions and recommend them highly to other theological schools for serious consideration."

In his chapter, Granger noted that without critical reflection, seminaries in the United States had adopted the didactic European form of theological education, continuing "the college pattern of classroom lectures, note-taking, examination-passing, and fraternity-like life without linking the courses to the real world and without expecting the student to assume more responsibilities than he had in college." A few seminaries had internship years, but, said Granger, "the intern year resembles unsupervised fieldwork much more than clinical theological education. The student is very much on his own, and the insights he gains occur almost accidentally."

Granger proposed not just tinkering with the curriculum but transforming it: "I would like to see a few seminaries experiment with a completely revised approach to theological education in which the practical and the theoretical would be so inextricably bound together that at almost no point in the seminary curriculum would they be separated."

Granger acknowledged that he was learning a lot from the medical education model in which "professors and students go back and forth between classroom and clinic, theory and practice":

It has been inspiring to watch a medical professor, who is both an outstanding scholar and clinician, as he finishes his lecture of a highly theoretical subject and then invites his students to make rounds with him to demonstrate immediately the clinical implications of his theory …

It is difficult for a clergyman to visualize his former professor of systematic theology finishing a lecture and then going out into the clinic, a nearby church, to demonstrate the clinical implications of the doctrines he has been expounding. Such a thought is almost ludicrous.

Following are some of the elements of Granger's proposal.

1. Students would have supervised clinical experiences throughout their four years in seminary.
2. The students' clinical experiences would be as concurrent as possible with classroom teaching.
3. Churches located near the seminary would be the main "clinical classrooms." Pastors of the churches in which students would be placed would serve as community-based clinical instructors.
4. The clinical instructors would have weekly conferences with individual students. They would observe students at work and help them critique their work, sometimes by reviewing tapes of their teaching or other activities.
5. Students and their clinical instructors would meet for twice-weekly seminars in which they would use the case study approach, role-playing, and other techniques. From time to time seminary professors would sit in on discussions.
6. In addition to churches, the "clinical classrooms" could include such settings as college campuses, social agencies, homes for the aged, hospitals and prisons. If these institutions were at a great distance from the seminary, students would have an intensive supervised clinical experience and then return to the seminary.

At the time Granger wrote this proposal, students entering traditional, mainstream seminaries needed to have a bachelor-level degree. Then, after three or four years in seminary, they received a bachelor's degree in divinity (BD). Granger argued that seminarians in mainstream seminaries were doing graduate level work and so should be rewarded with a graduate-level degree.

Healing in Congregations

In addition to wanting to transform theological education, Granger was excited about what he saw as the enormous potential for healing within congregations. The ideas he presented in a sermon in 1960, which he gave both at Rockefeller Chapel and Beloit College Chapel, were seed ideas for the roles that lay people would play in the Wholistic Health Centers that Granger created a decade later. The sermon was based on Luke 9:2: "And he [Jesus] sent them out to preach the kingdom of God and to heal." Granger said: "There is a magnificent rebellion against a religion that only preaches and fails to heal." Preaching and teaching is not the minister's task alone. Nor is healing restricted only to physicians.

It is "entirely probable," said Granger, that properly educated Christian lay people "can provide a quality and range of care beyond anything ever imagined." They can provide "pastoral healing of troubled individuals as well as the healing of troubled homes."

In another talk[14] Granger again presented ideas that sounded like the future Wholistic Health Centers. "Church buildings stand vacant a large part of the week." Instead, Granger proposed that during the week, some of the space could be used for a clinic, for counseling services, or for "day-hospitals" where people in distress could come for pastoral care and other services. Therapy groups of various sorts could be conducted. Services could be related to an individual church or to a council of churches. People representing religion, social work, and medicine could provide the services. Granger spoke also of how lay people could contribute. Alcoholics Anonymous, he said, has demonstrated that concerned fellow sufferers can be of help to each other. Lay people in the church can also be trained to help pastors with their heavy counseling loads.

Granger continued to talk about the church as a potential place of healing. A few years later, speaking to a group of pastors,[15] he said, "I think of the church as more than a building that is open on Sunday morning and for an occasional meeting during the week. I see the church as a potential meeting place for people who are concerned about the total health of the people in their community."

Granger said that he wanted people who are in trouble, even in emotional trouble or grieving, to feel welcomed into the church. He suggested that churches could serve their communities by inviting mental health clinics to use their facilities. The church could have a director of volunteers who could find people who would be willing to set up activities at the church that would be responsive to the needs of people who came to the clinic. As some troubled people began feeling better, Granger said the director of volunteers might also help them serve others as a way to continue healing themselves.

The more deeply Granger considered factors contributing to the troubles the people might bring to their encounters with both the church and medical professionals, the more his thoughts turned to the power of grief to disturb well-being. If the church was to be a partner in healing perhaps it needed a fuller understanding of how illness comes about—including the role of grief in some illness. This topic grew into a major interest of Granger's lifelong campaign to support and treat the whole person.

Connecting Ministers and Doctors in the Care of People

Granger was still eager to bring clergy and physicians together around the care of people. In the summer of 1959, when he went to Union Seminary to teach a course on religion and health with his brother-in-law, Daniel Day Williams, Granger hoped to make progress on the manuscript that he eventually titled *Minister and Doctor Meet*. Granger took 18-year-old Jane with him because she had been working with him on the book, and he wanted her continued help. Granger was also eager to get Lael's feedback.

Granger divided the manuscript into four parts.

1. The Patient: Focus of Doctor and Minister

2. How the Minister Functions in the Sickroom
3. Psychiatry as it Relates to Minister and Doctor
4. Areas of Joint Concern for the Minister and Doctor

Lael reviewed what Granger wrote. Among other things, she questioned the conversational style of the writing. She thought the book should be couched in more academic language. Granger, however, wanted the book to be accessible to all readers, not just academics. He never saw himself as an intellectual and never pretended to be one.

After returning from his few weeks in New York, Granger and Jane continued working on the manuscript of *Minister and Doctor Meet*. Several months later, Granger submitted the first draft to Harper & Row. Granger: "They accepted the manuscript but said I had spelled 'wholistically' incorrectly, that I should drop the w. I wrote them a nice long letter saying, please let me spell it with a w. It will make it easier for people to understand the concept of wholeness. They agreed to this. Years later I was pleased to open a dictionary and find that you can now spell 'wholistic' with a *w*."

Granger dedicated the book to Jane, writing,

To my eighteen-year old daughter Jane who
encouraged me to finish this book
gave up her summer vacation to type and retype the manuscript
made many suggestions regarding both style and content
which I heeded
daily gives me reason to have confidence in today's youth

In his review of *Minister and Doctor Meet* in 1961, Seward Hiltner wrote:[16] "By reporting and evaluating the very things in which his experience is most authoritative, Westberg has made a significant contribution to the ideas in this field. We always knew he was warm, human, and pastoral. We now know also that he can generalize his experience usefully for others, both ministers and doctors."

Orville S. Walters (a minister and a psychiatrist), then director of health services and lecturer in psychiatry at the University of Illinois, included the following in his review:[17]

> In contrast to many of the eager books on pastoral care that have deluged the market recently, this one has come to maturity over a period of 20 years, during which the author has been an acknowledged leader in the movement for collaboration between clergyman and physician.
>
> … While recognizing the beneficial impact of dynamic psychiatry upon the ministry, Westberg has refrained from embracing the currently popular psychoanalytic psychology … While some in the field have achieved a reconciliation between religion and the sciences by trimming theology to fit a naturalistic psychology, Westberg has qualified his acceptance of the new psychology by reaffirming a clear theological position. In this context he offers well-proven guidance to the clergyman who desires to minister effectively to the sick and to collaborate increasingly with the physician.

Walter Alvarez, then editor-in-chief of *Modern Medicine*, wrote: "Granger Westberg's book is essential for every minister and invaluable for doctors. Drawing on years of experience, an able and understanding hospital chaplain tells how to visit the sick and deal helpfully with their psychic problems."

Wayne Oates, professor of psychology of religion at Southern Baptist Seminary, wrote:[18] "This man writes from the boundary regions between the two professions where he works every day as an active teacher of both doctors and ministers. He does not just have the status. He does the work. No minister should miss this book."

Minister and Doctor Meet was generally well regarded but the chapter on grief was given the most attention.

Chapter 11

Good Grief

As a member of the staff of Rockefeller Memorial Chapel at the University of Chicago, Granger sometimes led the worship service at the chapel on Sunday mornings. This meant he got to interact with distinguished guest preachers. Granger: "At Rockefeller, I got to hear many remarkable people, including Reinhold and Richard Niebuhr, Albert Schweitzer, and the great theologian, Paul Tillich. I remember how nervous Tillich was before he preached. He said that he didn't think that he had anything worthwhile to say."

At least once a year Granger was asked to preach. His sermons, like others given at the chapel, were broadcast over WGN, a local Chicago radio station. Granger:

> On a typical Sunday when I would preach, I would get anywhere from 10 to 25 letters asking for copies of the sermon. That is, until the Sunday I preached on grief and health [March 5, 1961]. For that sermon we received almost 1,000 letters! I couldn't believe what had happened. I figured I had suddenly become a great preacher because even Paul Tillich, the Niebuhrs, and Harry Emerson Fosdick didn't get more than 300 letters. So I worked very hard on my next sermon (not related to grief) and waited for the avalanche of letters. I got about 12 letters.
>
> I decided that the topic of grief was of tremendous interest to all kinds of people.

In his sermon and in his chapter on grief in *Minister and Doctor Meet*, Granger drew on his decades of working with patients and their families and his longtime interest in grief that was sparked by the work of Harvard psychiatrist, Erich Lindemann.[1]

Granger described 10 stages that people typically appeared to go through as part of the grief process. He noted that no two people went through the process in the exact same way, but there appeared to be a pattern. Initially Granger had focused on grief following the death of a loved one or someone who had an important impact on the bereaved person's life. But very soon he realized that he observed the same stages in people who suffered other kinds of loss, such as the loss of a job and the loss of a child in marriage.

Granger wanted grieving people to know that they were not alone; that grief was a natural, even ultimately a growth-promoting, process, particularly "if we move through it with the help of our faith and the supporting concern of those around us." Granger also pointed out that getting stuck in one of the stages of the grief process can be unhealthy.

Granger identified the following stages of grief:

1. Shock
2. Emotional release
3. Depression and isolation
4. Physical symptoms of distress
5. Preoccupation with the loss that can lead to panic over the fear that we are going through something abnormal
6. Sense of guilt about the loss
7. Anger, hostility and resentment
8. Difficulty returning to usual activities
9. Gradual dawning of hope
10. Readjustment to reality

Granger's sermon on grief and "The Grief Process and Health" chapter in *Minister and Doctor Meet* touched people deeply. Some wrote that the grief they were experiencing following the loss of important people and things caused them to feel they were going crazy or that they would never recover from their deep despair. It was comforting, they said, to learn that Granger was able to describe a grieving process that had some important parallels to the process they were experiencing.

Granger received so many letters of gratitude that friends encouraged him to elaborate further on the stages of grief in a small book for laypeople. Granger proceeded with this task. On Helen's recommendation, he titled the resulting small book, *Good Grief.*[2]

After all of the positive feedback, Granger hadn't anticipated that it would be difficult to find a publisher. He first approached Harpers, the publishers of *Minister and Doctor Meet*, but, he recalled, "They didn't think it would sell. Then I tried our church press. Their first response was that they didn't think it would sell, so I wrote them a strong letter and talked to a few people on the board of directors. Finally they agreed to give it a try."

Good Grief got excellent reviews both from professionals in the field and from newspaper columnists. Mary Merryfield, who had a nationally syndicated advice column, wrote that when she heard Granger interviewed on television, she hurried out and got his book, which she then referred readers to in several of her columns. Walter Alvarez, the surgeon with a nationally syndicated column, wrote that he thought the book would be "very helpful to thousands of grief-stricken people."

The Westberg children had fun with *Good Grief*. Charles Schultz had published a book of his comic strips called *Good Grief, Charlie Brown.*[3] In Schultz' comic strip, a familiar refrain was "Good Grief, Charlie Brown." Granger's children would go into bookstores, find the two books, and put them together on a shelf.

By 1987, *Good Grief* had sold one million copies. Over the years almost every time Granger spoke in public, people would approach him afterward and tell him how much *Good Grief* had helped them during a time of great loss. Pastors, nurses, physicians, funeral directors, and even veterinarians gave *Good Grief* to patients and clients. Granger received thousands of letters of thanks. One was from Mamie Eisenhower, who wrote that after husband "Ike" (President Dwight D. Eisenhower) died, a friend had given her *Good Grief* and the book had helped her deal with her grief. Another woman said that when her sister died, her parents sent out 350 copies of *Good Grief* to their friends instead of Christmas cards. "Compassionate Friends," a self-help group of parents and siblings grieving the loss of a child/sibling wrote that *Good Grief* was almost like a Bible for their group.

A couple wrote that *Good Grief* was of great help when their oldest child was killed in a car accident. "*Good Grief* guided and reassured us through the months and years of our grief, not unlike the guidance and reassurance we got by reading Dr. Spock's books during the early years of child rearing. We have bought dozens of copies of *Good Grief* through the years to comfort friends who were grieving. Everyone has appreciated the gift," they said.

"Good grieving," Granger wrote in one of the later editions of *Good Grief*, could help people mature.[4] "If we were to draw a line describing growth toward maturity," he said, "it probably would not be a straight line moving gradually upward." Rather the line would go up and down like a roller coaster. There would be "little dips, middle-size dips, and big dips."

> The little dips are the smaller kinds of problems or grief with which all of us struggle on almost a daily basis. These dips may take anywhere from a few hours to a few days to work through. We usually handle them by ourselves, with close friends ... How people handle little dips has much to say about how they will probably handle bigger dips, so it is important that we understand that many of the same dynamics are present in all three sizes of dips.

Granger described each dip as having three stages—plateau, dip, and thrust. Life can be going along smoothly on a plateau when suddenly something comes along that puts you into a dip. If you deal successfully with the dip, you may actually thrust up to a higher level before leveling off into another plateau. This kind of growth, he noted, is not restricted to responses to a loss or negative event. It can occur when one faces all kinds of challenges.

In 2011 the fiftieth anniversary edition of *Good Grief* included the following foreword by Dr. Timothy Johnson, then ABC News senior medical contributor:

> I just finished rereading this gem. It is immediately clear that it has been, and will continue to be, a best seller. It is written with the heart of a pastor, the insight of a psychologist, the humanity of a father and husband, and the hope of someone who has seen so many survive the process of grieving. It is simple but not simplistic. It is profound but not professorial. More importantly, it describes the pathway through grieving that can only be found through honesty. This is a book that should be in the hands of anyone grieving for any reason.

In early 1961, the same year Granger first preached on "good grief" in Rockefeller Chapel, he had to face the grave illness of his beloved sister, Viola. Two years earlier Viola and her husband had moved to Antioch, California, where her husband, Roger, had accepted a call as pastor of a small Lutheran church. The move was very difficult for Viola. When she became ill, Granger contacted his surgeon friend, Garrett Allen, who had been at the University of Chicago but was now at Stanford University. Allen operated and found that Viola had cancer that was so widespread that there was nothing the medical team could do.

When *Good Grief* was published, Granger dedicated it "to the memory of my sister, Viola, who helped so many find hope in the midst of grief." This dedication was translated into many other languages as *Good Grief* was published internationally.

Months after Viola's death, in a paper Granger presented at the 1961 Annual Meeting of the American Cancer Society, he noted that grief reactions often take place "not only in patients but to some degree in all those persons who are near to them." The symptoms, he said, "are just about the same" in patients and relatives.

> We have found that we are able to help these people face their anticipated or actual loss by encouraging them to wrestle openly and honestly with questions that such grief raises. We seek to help them "work through" their grief in a permissive relationship where they can question all their former beliefs about God and rethink the basic philosophy on which their whole life is built.

The Lutherans' Grief Process

For some time, the Augustana Lutheran Church in which Granger grew up and served as a pastor had struggled with its future. Now members of Augustana Lutheran Church were going through an overt "good grief" process. In 1962 the Augustana Lutheran Church had decided to give up its separate identity and merge with three other Lutheran church bodies. The church's 103rd and final convention was a time of grieving for people who were still tightly linked to the past, but it was an exciting day for Granger and others who were eager to move forward.

The convention included the ordination service for the last class of Augustana seminarians, including Jane's first husband, Don Olson. The sign of ordination, the stole, is placed on the seminarian by his pastor or someone else who is close to him. Granger placed the stole on Don.

The next morning the presidents of the four church bodies[5] stepped to a microphone and read identical statements affirming the consolidating action of their churches. After the statements were read, the chairman of the constituting convention, Malvin Lundeen, declared that the Lutheran Church in America was duly constituted.[6]

The merger of the four Lutheran church bodies into one church now led to the need for a new seminary. In September 1962, the Lutheran School of Theology at Chicago (LSTC) was established as a consolidation of four seminaries.[7] The move to unity opened the door at last to the Lutheran presence Granger had long wanted on the University of Chicago campus.

Clergy and Physicians Down Under

The success of Granger's work was leading to more and more invitations for him to speak. In the summer of 1963, medical and religious societies of Australia and New Zealand invited Granger to spend a month talking with groups of clergy and physicians about wholistic health and some of the ways in which clergy and physicians in the United States were beginning to work together.

Helen, who had stayed home while Granger made countless trips over the years, finally got to travel with Granger on a trip that circled the globe. Helen: "First we had a little time for visiting in Europe. In Australia and New Zealand everyone was extremely friendly, but they really pushed Granger. He had to work day and night, giving talks, appearing on radio shows, and all. We finally had to ask that he be given time off so that he could have a haircut, but even then they sent him with someone who needed counseling. So he worked the whole time."

The haircut apparently made quite a hit. In Melborne, Neil Jillet, a newspaper journalist, described Granger this way:[8] "Dr. Westberg has a crewcut, an enviable tan and the cheery good looks of the all-American boy. He is aged 50 and could easily be mistaken for younger than 40."

Granger recalled, "Following my presentations I was deeply impressed with the quality of the questions raised by clergy and physicians. I was impressed with the dedication of the physicians. Most of them did not seem to make as much money as US physicians did, and many seemed to be active in their churches. Months and years after the trip, I was very pleased to hear that following the meetings, clergy and physicians started talking and working more together."

Chapter 12

Raising the Curtain on Three Acts of Illness

Since he first became a chaplain at Augustana Hospital in 1944, Granger, with likeminded colleagues, worked toward more general acknowledgement of the importance of chaplains and toward raising their professional standards. In 1959 the American Hospital Association (AHA) created a committee on chaplaincy services that Granger was invited to chair. The committee created a document first titled "Outlines of a Chaplaincy Program," which eventually became a manual: *Essentials of a Hospital Chaplaincy Program*. Granger said,[1] "This was the first official document published by the AHA indicating to its member institutions that pastoral care of patients was to be encouraged in all hospitals of the country whether affiliated with religious groups or not."

In 1961 the American Medical Association (AMA) acknowledged the importance of the spiritual dimension of health care by creating a department of medicine and religion, which in time was headed by a full-time clergy person, Paul B. McCLeave. Closely related to this department was a committee made up of 15 clergy, each from a different denomination. Granger was on this committee for 10 years.

In December 1963 the AHA and AMA jointly sponsored a Special Invitational Conference on Hospital Chaplaincy. In his opening address to the audience of Protestant, Catholic, and Jewish clergy, Granger said:[2]

We have come to a challenging moment in the development of the hospital chaplaincy movement. During the past 25 years we have watched it grow from small beginnings with a very few elderly men, who were only tolerated in a hospital setting, to a group numbering in the hundreds, including men of all ages, who have had anywhere from three months to three years of specialized training.

That the chaplaincy program is now being taken seriously by leaders in medicine and health care is attested to by our being invited by the American Hospital Association and the American Medical Association to gather for this period of two days. It is significant that a meeting such as this one would, in all probability, not have been called by the AHA and AMA only two or three years ago.

Granger suggested two possible reasons that the AHA and the AMA had kept the medical and religious aspects of health care separate. First, they were reluctant to get involved in the problems between various religious groups, and second, they did not believe that "the religious dimension was of any real significance in the scientific care of people who are ill." Granger said that the first concern was being addressed by the successful ecumenical movement—first among Protestants and more recently among Protestants, Catholics, and Jews. Regarding the second concern, the work of clinically educated chaplains over the past 25 years was apparently helping to convince some physicians and administrators that the religious dimension was worthy of recognition.

However, Granger said that chaplains still faced many challenges. Speaking at a time when the large majority of chaplains were men and the language was still not gender sensitive, Granger said:[3]

The first glow of enthusiasm about the chaplain's presence in the hospital is now waning. He must prove his worth, just as any other member of a helping profession, and this will not be easy because of the scientific criteria that will be used to judge the effectiveness of his work. In the past he has done his share of criticizing the inadequacy of an atomistic approach to patient care and has preached his share of sermons on the value of the wholistic approach. Now as the hospital chaplain matures and begins to evaluate his own work, he is frank to say that he isn't doing as much for patients as he had hoped to do, and he sees that he has only begun what he hopes will develop into a more effective spiritual ministry.

Granger sounded a theme that he was to pursue in the coming years. He expressed gratitude to the psychiatrists, social workers and psychologists who had helped provide clinical pastoral education, but he expressed concern that theological students were not clear about their identity and role because some of their non-clergy teachers were not sure about the role of clergy in health care, particularly the theological dimensions.

Illness in Three Acts

When doing chalk talks for lay people, Granger likened the progression of illness to the three acts of a play.⁴ With a smile, he would say, "The technical name for what goes on in Act 1 is 'a little-bit sick.' The name of Act 2 is 'sicker,' and the title for Act 3 is 'really sick.'"

Although the three acts were somewhat simplistic, even quaint, they were fresh and important in their time. As the years went by, Granger updated his talk so it was more in alignment with the growing understandings about health maintenance and disease prevention. Granger:

In Act 1, you are cruising along through life, working hard, attending daily to the stream of obligations and joys with which you surround yourself, and you begin to notice a nagging sense that everything is not right. The first person to notice that you are sick may be you. You suddenly realize that you don't feel so good. You're a little bit sick.

Then you begin to try to figure out what's going on. You act as your own doctor, listen to the symptoms, and make a diagnosis. You may decide that you've been burning the candle at both ends and not getting enough sleep. Your fatigue and headache are the first signs that you're not getting away with this pace unscathed. So you decide on a treatment: "Every night for the next five nights, I'm going to bed at 10 o'clock. Then I'll see what happens." You treat yourself. If your diagnosis was accurate, based on your knowledge of yourself, and if you do follow your treatment plan, then probably you'll get well again.

Most of us do this all of the time. We go in and out of Act 1 continually, constantly adjusting our schedule, pace, and ways of taking care of ourselves in light of the feedback our own systems provide us.

But, let's say you don't listen to yourself and your feedback. You keep pressing on, working too hard. You may get sicker. One of your children says, "Hey Dad, is something wrong? You don't look well, and you've sure been a grouch." You reply, "No, nothing's wrong. I am not irritable. *I am not irritable!*" But if you listen to your family's feedback, acting as your doctor, you may decide to change your pace and get yourself well again.

You discover that you're in Act 2 of illness when you realize that you're sick enough that you need to do something right now. You call your family's physician and see him or her as soon as possible. Let's say he's the listening kind and he listens to your problem. Then he examines you and together you sit down and talk. "You know," he says, "Your fatigue and headaches appear to be related to the stress you're under. What can we do to help you make some changes in your lifestyle?"

If you listen to him, and the two of you decide on ways to lessen your stress, you probably will move out of Act 2, through Act 1, and get well again. If the treatment you and your doctor decide on doesn't work, or if you don't follow his advice, you may go back three or four times for the same problem. Finally, he may say. "I think you'd better come into the hospital for a checkup." So you go into your community hospital for a checkup, which may include x-rays, extensive laboratory work, perhaps even exploratory surgery. Then another diagnosis and treatment plan are made, and you get well again.

Many people go through a large portion of life seldom getting sicker than this. Thus the family physician can take care of almost all health problems you experience throughout life.

A small percentage of us, however, get sicker than Act 2, and move into Act 3. The family physician finally doesn't know what to try next. He feels he can't handle the problem any longer and says, "I'd like you to see a friend of mine who is a specialist."

Now you see the specialist. The specialist is able to recognize and deal with your problem because it's big now, and because he knows this particular type of problem very well. Occasionally, he says, "I think you'd better come to the hospital." So you go to the research and teaching hospital, and there you see not just specialists but a super-specialist or a sub-specialist. The specialists and sub-specialists on your case put their collective heads together and do some remarkable work with your disease, and you get sent back to your family doctor, and then to your friends and family, and you get well again.

At the far end of Act 3 looms Act 4, the realm of undertakers and ministers. Most of us spend our lives trying to stay out of this act.

Granger pointed out that during any given day, most people are in Act 1 and very few people are in Act 3. However, most physicians focus on the later stages of illness. Optimistically Granger said that he thought there was a trend for professionals to move into earlier stages of illness and prevention. As part of keeping people out of Acts 2 and 3 as much as possible, he pressed to involve the resources of the church, including transforming theological education.

Granger himself was eager to spend more time working with people who were in Act 1. Although he had great appreciation for the role of clergy in the hospital, during his last years at the University of Chicago, he was growing restless with this role for himself: "I had no regrets for the years I spent doing the best job I could but I wasn't satisfied doing this the rest of my life." Granger said that his experiences in dealing with hundreds of very sick people "forced me to decide that someday I would like to get into one of the earlier acts or stages of illness where my expertise as a pastor could possibly help to reverse the process and keep people from getting sicker. I was particularly interested to see how clergy could be helpful to people who were going through grief or other stressful situations."

A Proposal Before Its Time

For many years Granger had tried to convince the faculty of the Divinity School to explore some of the ideas for radically changing theological education that he had proposed in his 44-month plan in the late 1950s. These ideas included more involvement of seminarians in Act 1. In early 1964 he wrote a proposal to the curriculum committee of the Divinity School about the expansion opportunities for his Office of Medicine and Religion in the university. In his proposal he pulled together several of the ideas he had been describing over the years, along with his optimism generated by the successful AMA and AHA-sponsored conference for chaplains.

Granger: "During the next five to 10 years, scores of hospitals will not only establish chaplain's departments but will also desire chaplains who are qualified to teach theological students and to participate in the teaching of medical students and residents. As we see it, the demand will far exceed the supply of chaplains unless schools like the University of Chicago take seriously the training of exceptionally qualified chaplains who can provide leadership for the future development of medicine and religion."

Granger proposed that the University of Chicago continue to take the lead in preparing highly qualified chaplains and in motivating other universities to establish solid programs. Among other things, he proposed that during the next 10 years his Office of Medicine and Religion (at that time comprised of himself and a part-time secretary) take on projects including:

1. Research in the area of grief as a precipitator of illness.
2. Creation of an out-patient pastoral counseling clinic, which would have a close relationship with the departments of psychiatry and social work, and which would, among other things, help clarify the areas of cooperation between religion, psychiatry and social work.
3. Establishing, in a nearby church, an experimental clinical training center patterned on present hospital clinical training centers for clergy.

Granger was pleased that students were having clinical pastoral care experiences in the hospital, but he also wanted them to be exposed to people in the early, more reversible, stages of illness.

Granger also contended that seminary graduates deserved a graduate level degree. This degree, he argued again as he had in his original proposal, might help physicians and other professionals treat clergy more as equal colleagues.

The curriculum committee voted down Granger's ideas.

Experiencing a Big Dip

Understandably, Granger was discouraged, and this state of mind converged with an unexpected, intriguing opportunity.

> I wasn't getting any place with my ideas. My colleagues weren't ready to change things in the Divinity School, and I was feeling discouraged. Then out of the blue, about a week after my ideas had been voted down by the curriculum committee, Dawson Bryan, who had established the Institute for Religion in Houston, Texas, visited me. For the past eight or nine years I had watched with interest what had been taking place in Houston, and I had participated, from time to time, in some committee deliberations. Dawson was a delightful, soft-spoken man who had been pastor of a huge Methodist Church. He had great zeal for getting pastors in touch with the medical world and had raised money for the creation of the Institute of Religion, a center for clinical pastoral education, located in the heart of the medical center. After we visited for a while, he invited me to be the Dean of the Institute. Naturally because of my discouragement with my own university, I was in the mood to do something different. I accepted the invitation.

Granger's level of discouragement must have been deep, indeed, because he gave up a position at a major university that included his unique appointment in the schools of theology and medicine, including tenure.

Three months after Granger accepted the deanship of the Institute, but while he was still at the University of Chicago, the membership of curriculum committee at the University of Chicago changed. The new committee voted to give the MDiv degree and took some of Granger's other ideas, though they were presented in a different style. "If I could have stayed," Granger reflected later, "I think I could have accomplished something. It made me sick to think that I was leaving a place where we could have developed a program that the whole country would have observed. That put me in a very depressed state. It took me months to get over that."

As Granger was preparing to leave the University of Chicago, he received the following letter from H. Stanley Bennett, dean of the biological sciences, University of Chicago:[5]

> We have watched with admiration the development of your splendid work here. You have recognized the community of purpose and opportunities for joint service which clergymen and physicians share and have developed practical skills in implementing an effective collaboration, not only locally, but on a national—and indeed, international—scale. Your talents in pastoral work, in scholarship, in administration, and in promotion have borne forth great fruit and have earned the gratitude of our institution, our administrators, and of physicians throughout the world.

Around this time, the following comment was made in the "Notes and News" section of *Pastoral Psychology*:[6] "Seward Hiltner has written that 'imaginative exploration of new dimensions—of ministry, of teaching, and of study—are thoroughly characteristic of Granger Westberg.' Surveying Westberg's achievements, one may venture an educated guess that he will continue pioneering ventures in clinical pastoral education in Houston."

Chapter 13

The Living Human Document

As dean of the Institute of Religion (now the Institute for Spirituality and Health) in Houston, Texas, Granger's academic appointment was professor of medicine and religion in the department of psychiatry of Baylor College of Medicine. The Institute and the medical school are located in the heart of the Texas Medical Center in Houston. Dawson Bryan had been president of the Institute since its beginnings in 1954.

The Institute of Religion brought together five Texas seminaries in a graduate program of pastoral care and counseling."[1, 2] A three-month course for pastors and theological students focused on "pastoral care of the sick and the afflicted." A one-year graduate internship in pastoral care and counseling prepared ministers for "better pastoral ministry, for hospital chaplaincy and for advanced graduate clinical study." A second-year residency provided specialized training for ministers who wanted to become clinical theological educators. Annually a postgraduate course in family counseling and the care of the sick and bereaved was held for pastors in the Houston area. The affiliated seminaries awarded credit toward the bachelor of divinity degree and master's and doctoral degrees.[3]

Granger was impatient to get going on a new project. Before moving to Houston, Granger, Helen, Joan and Jill had spent two weeks in August at College Camp on Lake Geneva. But it was cold, so Granger called Dawson Bryan to see if they could come early.

A bewildered Dawson, in the throes of a hot and humid Houston summer, said to come ahead.

Helen and Granger had already picked out their home in a lovely wooded community with three little lakes. When the family arrived in Houston, Dawson and Rachel Bryan helped Granger and Helen get acquainted and feel at home by hosting dinners and luncheons.

In early September 16-year-old Joan entered her junior year in a local high school. Jill, age 10, began fifth grade. John remained in La Grange. With his new position as superintendent of Oakridge Cemetery and his many friends, he was ready to be on his own. Jane and Don were at their first church in Hialeah, Florida, with their seven-month-old son, Brian—Granger and Helen's first grandchild.

In Granger's address at the Baylor Medical School Convocation that fall, he described the Institute as "an unusual experiment in clinical theology that could ultimately change the nature of the church or synagogue you attend." He also said that it was a "unique experiment in graduate theological education that is calling into question the traditional methods of teaching and preparing people for the ministry." Further, he said:

> It is a new, vital, ecumenical institute that is not fettered by particular denominational ties that tend to say, 'We have taught theology this way for 400 years, and we plan to continue to do it this way.' It is the only institute dedicated to a dialogue between religion and the health sciences with a building and a faculty located in the middle of a dynamic medical center.

Granger continued:

> ... The Institute hopes to demonstrate that there are newer and better ways of making theology come alive. This can be done chiefly by helping students to become existentially involved in the world around them and to listen deeply to the

kinds of questions raised by people in all walks of life and in all human situations.

When he was in seminary, Granger said he and his classmates were told to "read, read, read." They tried but found that many books were "dull and stuffy."

> Our teachers had not yet discovered ways to first dunk us deeply in the waters of life so that we would come up gasping and questioning everything. Most of us had lived a protected life up to that point, and now we were being fed second-hand theology for four years in another protected environment.
>
> The Institute operates on the premise that the student should first be introduced to the "living human document" on the assumption that "life comes before literature." We have found that these students are then much more willing to take the library of books seriously because they have been motivated by their encounter with life itself.

Granger encouraged the audience of medical educators "to participate in the education of our clergy." He said, "When our students come over into the hospitals and clinics, as they do every day, engage them in discussion about their work. Ask them what they hope to do to help your patient ... Prod them a bit. Don't let them hide behind theological jargon."

As the new dean, Granger was eager to get to know all of the faculty members at the Institute and in the affiliated institutions. Julian Byrd, a faculty member based at M. D. Anderson Hospital, recalled:

> One of the things that stood out for me was how within a week or so after Granger came, he found out that I was doing the chapel service at M. D. Anderson Hospital. I was really touched that one of the first things that Granger, as the new dean, did was come out on Sunday to hear me conduct a worship service.

He even asked me for a copy of my sermon.

He made the rounds and visited all the faculty members. He established himself as someone who wanted to get to know the personalities of the people that were at the Institute. So we had a very pleasant working relationship.

Disrupted by a Brush with Death

Granger's plans to get to know the faculty, however, were derailed. He explained:

On September 15 I flew to Dallas to speak to the Dallas County Medical Society. When I returned to the airport that evening, I called Helen and told her that I was safely back. Then I picked up a little Volkswagen that belonged to one of the other teachers at the Institute. He had asked me to drive it to my home for him. The last thing I remember was going the speed limit of 45 miles per hour.

Later, the man who hit me came to the hospital and told me, "I had fallen asleep at the wheel. When I woke up, I found myself way on the left side of the road. There was no way I could miss hitting you. The only thing I could do was to head for the ditch."

The man who hit me was driving a big station wagon. I couldn't avoid him. My car was totaled.

Luckily a police car was only a few cars behind me. They got to us right away. I remember one of the policemen asking me, "What hospital do you want to go to?" I replied, "Methodist."[*] He said, "That's too far. There is a new hospital out here." I said, "Please, please take me to Methodist." When they asked me what doctor I wanted, all I could think of was Dr. DeBakey.[5]

When we got to Methodist Hospital, two of Dr. DeBakey's residents were the first ones to see me and checked me over. Helen came to see me, and then they suddenly took me into another room. One of the residents said, "We've got a problem. You're losing a lung. We're going to have to puncture you and put a tube in you. We hate to do this to you, but we really have to do it. It will hurt like heck." Soon after that, I heard someone saying, "The other lung is going too." And they had to do the other lung as well. All of this happened in the emergency room without benefit of an anesthetic. This was an interesting experience. I often wondered how things were before the days of anesthesia. But don't ask me! I may tell you.

Later I learned that the small hospital where the ambulance drivers had planned to take me had only one nurse available at that time. If I had gone there, I probably wouldn't have made it.

Helen gave her perspective:

Dawson Bryan called and told me that Granger had been in an accident. He said, "I'm afraid he's lost most of his teeth." When I got to hospital the first thing I did was look at Granger's mouth. I was relieved when I saw that he still had his teeth and there was no blood. Also, Granger was telling the doctors that he hoped it wouldn't be necessary to stay in the hospital because he had all kinds of things to do in his new job. So I thought Granger would be okay, and I wasn't overly concerned when they suddenly took him into another room. A little while later, Dawson hurried into the room where I was and said, "They just saved your husband's life." I was shocked because when I saw Granger, it hadn't looked like he was that badly hurt.

When John heard the news of his father's accident, he drove nonstop from Chicago to Houston to be with the family. He didn't tell them he was coming, so Helen was surprised the next day when she came home from the hospital, looked into the house through the big bay window, and saw John playing the grand piano. With exaggerated flourish, John was moving his hands around on the keyboard, looking as if he was playing a great concerto. This gave Helen a much-needed laugh. John had been very resistant to practicing the piano when he was a child and had seldom touched a piano since childhood.

Granger's left ankle and right knee were smashed, and he had multiple other injuries. Because of his collapsed lungs, surgery could not be done for a couple of weeks on his legs, which had been put in temporary casts. Granger, who was accustomed to having great energy and exuberance, was weak, in pain, and dependent upon the care of others. Having spent much of his career ministering to people in hospital beds, now Granger was the one in need. As he said, "I was getting some of my own medicine."

Granger had to meet most of his new colleagues while dressed in a hospital gown, lying flat on his back in his hospital bed—not a particularly auspicious way to begin his work. As he started mending, he was allowed to dress and move around. He took advantage of a tunnel between Methodist Hospital and the Institute and got various people to wheel him back and forth between his hospital bed and the Institute so he could begin working.

Hearing about Granger's accident, Jerald Brauer, dean of the Divinity School at the University of Chicago, wrote Granger saying: "The news of your injury proved how much you are still in the hearts and minds of your many colleagues and friends at The University of Chicago." When the faculty got the news, they were shocked and greatly distressed. Brauer continued:

> These men were not expressing the perfunctory concern that is common when news of a disaster is received. They were genuinely and deeply concerned about you. Probably a man never realizes how much impact he makes in a situation and on other human beings until an occasion like this arises. Let me assure you, Granger, that the love and the esteem of the men of the Divinity School for you, Helen, and your family runs very deep.

After three longs weeks in the hospital, when he was finally ready to go home, Granger wrote the following to his mother, Alma:

Mom, I am writing this from my wheelchair that looks just like yours except that I have one leg in a cast which sticks straight out in front of me and makes it difficult for me to scoot around as fast as you. I should take lessons from you ...

I was immensely impressed by what cards, letters, phone calls, flowers, and humorous toys can accomplish in raising the spirits of a person who is totally dependent upon other people for every single thing that keeps him alive and functioning. I have also come to attach new value to the personal voicing of a prayer in the presence of a sick person. I am sure that I have been erring on the side of not praying enough in sick rooms because I didn't want to "overdo the prayer business."

Now I'd rather err on the side of praying too often. Those days and nights are awfully long and I was glad to have 10 brief prayers every day. I found that in my weakened condition it was difficult to pray, and so I very much appreciated those who helped me to pray by formulating the words for me. I am already looking back on this whole experience as one that served a teaching function for me.

The healing process took a long time. Granger had many weeks of painful physical therapy and home exercises. Initially this independent man was dependent on Helen, Joan and Jill, for the activities of daily living. As is the case with many people who have undergone significant, life-threatening trauma, Granger was discouraged, and his spirits were low. Being confined to a wheel chair and moving only with great pain was difficult on a man who enjoyed being physically active. Being without his usual energy and spirit was even more difficult.

Granger was grateful for all of the concern showed by Dawson Bryan and the others at the Institute, but he was impatient to feel like himself again and get back to work. As a good Lutheran with an overly strong work ethic, he probably also felt guilty that it was taking him so long to recover. As a workaholic of sorts, who almost never took a vacation, and certainly never "loafed" when he did, not being productive was almost unbearable.

By Thanksgiving, Granger was walking on crutches and only using his wheel chair for long distances. He wrote a letter of gratitude to family and friends for cards and letters they sent: "I have read them over and over and have a new appreciation of how a friend's name on a card or letter can transport me from my own apprehensive thoughts to pleasant thoughts about you and your kindness in remembering me."

Granger reported that he had gone to Chicago with Helen on a business trip. "I got to see my mother who was recently 93 and sharp as a tack. Our grand meeting took place in the hall of the Home for the Aged—both of us in wheelchairs raced toward each other. She won. She's had more practice!"

He also reported that the Texas Medical Center had its official reception for him and Helen. "They had put it off for two months. The receiving line was arranged so that I could sit on a bar stool throughout the two hours as some 150 board members and their wives from 15 institutions on the campus came by. It was a thrilling occasion."

Many years after Granger had recovered from his accident, a former student of his from the University of Chicago, Robert Graham Kemper, asked Granger what advice he would give to pastors about making hospital visits. Granger replied:[6]

My chief minister was my wife, and she needed help too. When the chaplains took time to have coffee or lunch with her, she was much more able to help me. I am more and more of the opinion that when you have 300 patients in the hospital, you must remember that there are at least 300 close relatives who are as much in need of care as the patient in the hospital.

Granger also encouraged clergy to visit members of their church in their homes:

It's surprising how few visits people make once patients get home. I was home for a couple of months, unable to get around because I was in a wheelchair, and few people came to see me. Yet when I was in the hospital 15 people wanted to come every day.

In early 1965, nationally syndicated columnist, Mary Merrifield wrote[7] that in March, 1964 she had written a column on grief and quoted from *Good Grief*. She continued, "The piece received a larger response over a longer period of time than any other column I've done. So today I'm reprinting highlights from that column along with an excerpt from a letter just received from Dr. Westberg."

Part of Granger's letter that Mary quoted was as follows:

I had a near-fatal auto accident in September. I wanted you to know that the stages of grief a person goes through when his professional life is set back follow essentially the same 10 stages outlined in my paperback, *Good Grief*. However, my ability to minister to people going through just such a process of "dip followed by an upward thrust" should be improved. And thanks to you for the hundreds of responses I received as a result of your column on grief last spring.

Despite lingering pain and diminished energy, Granger got back to work. Every morning, he conducted two seminars: one on the interrelation of medicine and religion and the other on preventive medicine and the parish pastor. In the latter seminar, Granger helped students examine the new field of community psychiatry and how it related to the life of the parish.

In the afternoon Granger helped to oversee the students' clinical experiences. Students worked in hospitals where chaplain-supervisors mentored and supervised them. The students also saw clients in the Institute's counseling service. These counseling sessions were tape recorded so the students and supervisors could review and reflect on the students' work. In the evenings, students were "on call" in one of the hospitals.

To help students reflect on these clinical experiences, Granger set up Interdisciplinary Religion-Medicine Case Conferences, using the model he had used at the University of Chicago.

Back in the Swing of Things

A year after his arrival in Houston, in the address he gave after formally being installed as dean of the Institute of Religion, Granger argued that students should have many opportunities to learn in laboratory settings, such as hospitals, college campuses, social agencies, settlement houses, and retirement homes. Echoing a proposal he had made when he was at the University of Chicago, Granger called for using space in churches for community psychiatry.

Granger now said he was "back in the swing of things." In a letter written in the fall of 1965, he spoke of giving at least one speech every day and frequently visiting three of the seminaries affiliated with the Institute, where he worked at recruiting prospective students. None of the affiliated seminaries were located in Houston, so it was not easy for Granger to get together with faculty from these schools. (Two seminaries were in Austin, two were in Fort Worth, and one was in Dallas.)

Granger was also very active again in the American Medical Association Committee on Medicine and Religion, the American Hospital Association Committee on Hospital Chaplaincy, and other national organizations.

In Houston, because of the design of his position and the scope of work, Granger had much less contact with medical students and physicians than he had at the University of Chicago. He felt badly about his lack of contact with medical students because he continued to think that physicians were more likely to work collaboratively with clergy in the care of people if they were introduced to the concepts of wholism and a health team that included clergy early in their education.

Granger's appointment was in psychiatry. He found caring physicians in his department and in the medical school, but he felt that few physicians were excited about his ideas. The culture of the medical center in Houston was probably shaped, in part, by the presence of the world-famous surgeon, Michael DeBakey, whose pioneering work in heart transplantation drew many physicians and others to the medical center. In his 80s Granger remembered, "The attitude of the doctors at the medical center was pretty much that surgery was the great thing. They were not very interested in what I had to say."

Even though Granger did not feel that he accomplished what he wanted to with the medical community, others felt differently. Julian Byrd said[8]:

> Granger was very instrumental in establishing breakthroughs with the medical community. Historically one of the missions of the Institute had been to provide education for medical students and young physicians in religion and health, and there had been courses offered at Baylor College of Medicine. But they were only elective courses, and the number of students they reached was limited.
>
> Granger was highly motivated and came with a lot of experience lecturing to medical students and faculty. He immediately started relating to the faculty of the medical school and was able to establish relations with senior heads of

department in a way that was a new beachhead for the Institute. This made a significant difference. Not all the medical people agreed that there was an important link between religion and medicine, but Granger was able to stimulate a level of dialog that had not been there before.

For those of us young faculty who had limited years of experience, Granger provided a model for us and an inspirational challenge that enabled all of us to achieve a deeper level of relationship with the medical community. This has continued. And the religion-medicine case conferences have continued.

Granger's time in Houston brought many challenges. Generally, students had responded very positively to his lectures. But this was an era in which students were speaking up to the professors and other members of the "establishment." One morning things did not go as Granger had planned in a class in which he had been doing a series of lectures. Writing some years later, he recalled,[9]

I well remember the severe trauma I experienced one morning in 1965 as I was about to begin the tenth lecture in a course I was giving. One of the ablest students in the class raised his hand and said, "We have had a meeting and have decided to ask you not to give any more lectures in this course because we aren't learning anything. You left us back at about the fifth lecture, and we feel the need to go back over all that you have said and have a chance to discuss it informally on our own level. Would you be willing to be a discussion leader rather than a lecturer?"

I was stunned. I always thought that I lectured on their level. I prided myself on moving at the student's pace, not mine. It was a terrible blow to my self-image. It took me two years to get over it. I went though a deep grief experience, which I am happy to say turned out to be "good grief."

Granger was accustomed to being the one challenging others to make changes. Now his students were urging him to change. For over a decade Granger had been using some collaborative instructional strategies, such as case presentations and role-plays intermixed with discussion. Apparently though, in some classroom settings, he resorted to more traditional lecturing and was not sufficiently sensitive to the needs of his students. As a result of this "traumatic" encounter, Granger did make changes in his teaching style. Speaking not only of himself but also of other colleagues who went through a similar experience, Granger wrote:

> Now none of us wants to go back to the old ways of teaching because there is a new kind of exhilaration that comes with working alongside of these young friends of ours who demonstrate much greater capacity for mature reflection and scholarly work when treated as colleagues and co-workers.

Granger was glad that theological students at the Institute and in seminaries were being given opportunities to learn in hospitals. He, of course, was a longtime advocate for clinical pastoral education in the hospital. However, he worried because some theological students tended to "glamorize the hospital" and "deglamorize the parish." They were "using psychiatric and medical jargon and didn't have much good to say about pastors or parishes." Perhaps, Granger speculated, this happened because hospitals were primarily workshops for doctors, and chaplains were seldom the strongest personalities on the hospital staff. "The psychiatrist, not the clergyman, was held up as the model for students," said Granger.[10]

> Although we are indebted to the medical profession, particularly psychiatry, for taking theological students under their wing when seminaries weren't interested in clinical teaching, we now have a responsibility to rethink the heavy hospital emphasis in pastoral ministry to the sick.

The hospital is not necessarily the only place, or even the best place, where this cooperative approach to health can be carried on.

Granger argued that most healing takes place in the home environment. He noted that the clergy are the only remaining members of the helping profession who have easy access to patients in their homes.

Granger tested the notion of having students spend time in a parish by asking some clinical pastoral education students to make home calls as assistants to the pastor of a local Methodist congregation of about 2,000 members. Initially the students resisted making calls. However, in their write-ups some students, particularly older graduates with parish experiences, said that as a result of what they had been learning in their courses they found themselves hearing and seeing things that they had missed when making house calls in the past.

The pilot project was working well, so with the pastor's encouragement, Granger arranged for the students to spend 15 to 20 hours a week at the church. The students did some teaching, helped with the worship service, and occasionally preached. Tape recordings were made of the students' teaching, and the pastor of the church spent one hour a week with each student in a supervisory session. Like the other students at the Institute, the seminarians who did clinical work in the parish spent five mornings a week at the Institute. They spent less time in hospitals than their counterparts.

Granger pointed to some of the advantages of this pilot program.

1. Almost immediately, the seminarians gained an identity as a "minister-to-be."
2. The students were in contact with a parish pastor who daily had a wholistic approach to people, which included their joys as well as their problems.
3. Because they made home calls in the community, the students

learned to minister to people in all kinds of conditions, including all stages of illness.

4. The presence of parish pastors on the Institute's teaching staff enriched the Institute.

After the course was completed, Granger wrote, "A number of the students became so interested in what a parish minister can do for the total health of the family that they stayed on with the pastor as volunteer assistants."

Despite these encouragements in his innovative work, Granger's Scandinavian blood did not seem to be suited for the South: "I couldn't believe what people in Houston go through in the summer. I would walk across the street from the Institute to Baylor Medical School. By the time I'd get there, I was wringing wet. I thought, 'Good night. I'm not going to live here.' Dawson was very kind and took us to a lake, but next to Lake Geneva, that lake was a depressing place." Granger also was having to take more responsibility for raising money, a job which he did not like and had not agreed to do.

Early in 1967, Granger and Helen went to Hawaii, where Granger did a five-day seminar. One day while they were sunning themselves on the beach, John Stump, the secretary for the Association of Lutheran Theological Seminaries, sat down to chat. Granger recalls that Stump asked, "Are you going to spend the rest of your life in the health field?" Granger replied, "I hope not." Stump explained that Hamma School of Theology was in need of a faculty member in practical theology. Stump asked Granger if he'd be willing to be a candidate.

Granger: "I felt guilty when I turned in my resignation. We stayed only three years and had some worthwhile experiences. But I didn't feel like I belonged."

Helen was not as convinced that it was time to leave Houston. She said, "I was very mixed. I felt that we hadn't yet finished."

After being in two high-powered medical centers—in Chicago and

Houston—Granger wrote,[11] "I decided to leave the highly specialized technology of a teaching and research hospital and move back into the community where people live and where one sees people in the earlier stages of illness—when illness is much more reversible. I also felt that as a minister my expertise lay chiefly in the area of preventive medicine."

As usual Granger was eager to get going. He hightailed it out of Houston as fast as he could. He let his youngest daughter, Jill, finish her last day of seventh grade—barely. Granger and Helen picked her up at school, and they left for Ohio from there.

Chapter 14

The Minister's Finest Hour

In his installation address at Hamma School of Theology, Wittenberg
University, in Springfield, Ohio, Granger said:[1]

> My appointment to Hamma School of Theology in Practical
> Theology and Continuing Education is a combination that
> makes sense to me, for if a clergyman desires to teach and to
> live theology that is practical, it is necessary that he continue his
> education the rest of his life. It is also true that every professor
> on this faculty is a professor of practical theology. This school
> happily does not tolerate professors of impractical theology.

When Granger arrived at Hamma, many of the students and
some of the faculty were unhappy with the typical lecture courses
offered by the seminary. The faculty invited Granger to talk with
them about his 44-month plan for theological education, which he
was glad to do. In *The Hamma Bulletin*, Roger Johnson, one of the
faculty members, wrote that in the fall of 1967, the Hamma faculty
adopted the substance of the Westberg proposal:

> They committed themselves to a professional education for the
> ministry, insisted upon the integration of theory and practice
> in all forms of learning, and developed an elaborate program
> of field education and supervision to realize this goal. They

also established the Master of Divinity as their basic degree. This differed from Westberg's proposal only in the respect that he had proposed a doctoral degree.

Changes in the Family

While Granger was helping to develop the new curriculum (putting some of his dreams into practice), Helen, Joan, and Jill were settling into Springfield, Ohio. Jill was in eighth grade. After one year at Augustana College, Joan transferred to Wittenberg University, where she majored in drama.

John had been drafted and was in Vietnam. As Granger wrote in a letter to Lael and Dan: "We live for his letters. Sometimes they make us happy, but most of the time they make us very blue. Yet there seems to be absolutely nothing we can do about the whole thing ... We never quite know what to do about listening to the news. Some days we can take it and other days we keep the radio and the TV turned off."

Jane and Don and their two sons were living in Miami. Don was associate pastor of a large Lutheran church, but the family lived in the parsonage of a dying church in a changing, unstable community. In the dying church, Don, with help from Jane and many others, created the Center for Dialogue, which included dialogues between what then was called the "establishment" and the "counter culture." Granger was interested in the free clinic that medical students set up in the Center for Dialogue. Dr. Lynn Carmichael, based at the University of Miami, was a pioneer in the evolving field of family medicine. He supervised the medical students at the free clinic. Some years later, to Granger's delight, Jane joined Carmichael and became a faculty member in the department of family medicine, which was home to the first family practice residency program in the US.

Apparently the proposed changes in the seminary curriculum did not happen as quickly as some of the students wanted. Perhaps the students were also emboldened by the student protests against the Vietnam War and for civil rights and free speech that were now occurring on campuses all over the nation, including the campus that Hamma shared with Wittenberg University. Granger recalled: "One older professor always left the room immediately after he gave his lecture. He didn't give students a chance to ask questions. One day a small group of students removed the platform, podium, and chairs from his classroom. In their place the students put beanbags. The poor old gentleman didn't know what to do."

Some professors did begin shifting from lectures to discussions. As students requested, some of the faculty invited students to call them by their first name. But, according to Granger, some professors had trouble with the transition. "They felt that these young people had so much to learn that they should be content to sit still and listen for at least two years before they should be allowed to express themselves."[2]

Not all of the students were pushing for change. Some students wanted things to remain the way they were. Granger said, "A number of students protested doing away with the lecture. They liked the structure that it gave and the ease with which they could take notes. They liked the feeling that there was an authority who knew what he was talking about. That felt good in a crazy, mixed-up world."

Years later, Carl Uehling, writing about the changes in Hamma's curriculum,[3] credited Granger with helping to design the new curriculum. Students, he said, now alternated between the classroom and six different internships, which were each up to three months long. Classes for new students began in June rather than October. Uehling reported that thanks to the curriculum, which gave students more responsibility, the use of library books was the highest in the school's history, and the book sales in the bookstore were "phenomenal."

Granger said that the church was having difficulty dealing with the challenges raised by the Vietnam War, the Civil Rights movement, the death-of-God controversy, the awareness of the deterioration of the inner cities, and the questioning of long-established institutions, including the church. Granger acknowledged that these were "some of the most difficult days the church has ever faced." Yet Granger saw possibilities for this being the minister's "finest hour."

At the installation of a pastor in February of 1968,[4] Granger said, "Ministers are baffled by the fast changing world about them. A few have given up the ministry in despair." In part, Granger contended, this might be due to the fact the church has been seen as "a preserver of the status quo ... of history and tradition." He continued, "The older way of teaching religion was to start with the distant past and then hope to finish the textbook by the time of graduation. But my profs never quite got us up to the present day. We spent most of our time in the sixteenth century. They seemed to have very little interest in the twentieth century."

One of the reasons that Granger saw this challenging time as potentially being one of the minister's finest hours was that more and more Christian people were reacting against the undue emphasis on a comfortable gospel. "While they appreciate the beauty of the worship service, the music, the Scriptures, the hymns, they know that this is only supposed to be preparation for the service to others that ought naturally to follow but often does not."

Both at the installation service and a later convocation service,[5] Granger spoke of how both Catholic and Protestant lay people all over the world are "coming awake," thanks, in part, to "an old man named Pope John XXIII, who was expected to serve only as an interim pope, but instead pulled the rug out from beneath the complacency of the Roman Catholic Church, and in so doing disturbed the complacency of Protestants as well."

Helen as Teacher Again

Some months after the family arrived in Ohio, a nun from St. Teresa's

School called Helen to see if she was interested in taking over for a fourth grade teacher who had to leave her teaching position because she "was in the family way." The nun said that some seminarians who had been doing a little substitute teaching knew about the opening and said that Helen might be interested in the position. They thought that since she had a son in Vietnam, she would probably welcome a distraction. Helen had missed teaching, and she did welcome the distraction, so she accepted the position.

In February 1968, Granger wrote in a family letter: "Helen's school teaching is the best thing that could have happened to her. She is becoming so attached to the children in her room and is discovering, I think, that she is a very good teacher—something she was never quite sure of when she taught 28 years ago at the orphanage where most of her work had to be disciplinary. These kids here in Springfield just love her. They even hang around after school to talk with her. You should have seen the handsome valentines she got."

That same month, John returned to the US to Fort Hood, Texas. Helen: "As soon as I heard from him, I put an American flag up outside. The neighbors all knew what this meant. John had been in Viet Nam for one year. He could have left a few weeks earlier, but he didn't want to leave his platoon in the lurch. The captain of his group had been wounded, and the new young lieutenant wasn't yet ready for major responsibilities. John stayed until he had trained someone to take his place."

The Parish Clergy

In 1963 during his last discouraging months at the University of Chicago, Granger managed to find energy to write a proposal, titled, "An American Academy of Parish Clergy: Why Not?" He had argued that the 250,000 parish ministers in the United States belonged to the only profession in the country without its own professional association to provide self-discipline, to support sustained growth, to study its own needs, and to strengthen the capacity of members to serve with effectiveness.[6]

According to Granger, the purpose of an academy was to encourage parish clergy of all faiths to spend approximately two weeks each year in some form of accredited continuing education "that will relate their religious faith to what is happening in the world around them." He proposed that the academy's services include the publication of an annual catalog of all continuing educational opportunities as well as a clearinghouse where clergy could learn about short-term courses available throughout the nation. He also said that academy staff would work both at convincing educational agencies, such as colleges and universities, to establish short-term courses for clergy and at convincing church organizations to release their clergy two weeks each year for continuing education.

In 1965, Granger's proposal was published in *The Christian Century*.[7] Clergy from all parts of the nation responded favorably to his proposal and urged that his suggestions be implemented. In response Granger wrote a proposal to the Lilly Endowment of Indianapolis, Indiana, requesting funding to establish an interdenominational, national Academy of Parish Clergy.

In 1968, Granger received a grant from the Lilly Foundation to establish the Academy. One of the first steps that Granger took in building the Academy was to bring together 20 parish pastors from 15 denominations. Granger got in touch with the presidents, bishops, and other heads of about a dozen denominations. He described the project and asked them to select one or two capable ministers who were interested in this issue and could meet with Granger and others. They did this. Granger: "I told them my dream. I said that I wasn't a parish pastor so I wouldn't tell them what to do. Also because I wasn't a parish pastor, I didn't feel I belonged in a leadership position in this group. I told them that I wanted to support their work, but I turned the organization over to them." Granger, however, did serve on the original board of the Academy.[8]

Reflecting on the meetings of the committee in Houston, Granger wrote,[9] "We are coming to see the parish clergyman as a "specialist" and the parish ministry as one of the important ministries of the church. The parish minister must stop being defensive. He must stop saying, 'I am only a parish pastor.' He must stop thinking that the parish church is on the way out and that his ministry will be of less and less value."

Just as the Academy of General Practice, with its requirement of continuing education courses, helped bring a sense of competence and self-worth to general practitioners of medicine, so, too, Granger predicted that the Academy of Parish Pastors, under the direction of accomplished parish pastors, could similarly bring new self-respect and competence to parish pastors.

Some months later, the editors of *The Christian Century* printed the following announcement:[10]

> One of the great joys of our work at *The Christian Century* is the unending flow of significant new ideas that come our way. It was just four years ago in our annual theological education issue for 1965 that Granger E. Westberg, then dean of the Institute of Religion at the Texas Medical Center in Houston, floated his proposal for an American Academy of Parish Clergy. Impressed by the continuing education program of general practitioners in medicine, Westberg pointed up the need for a professional association of parish ministers to develop standards of vocational competence and encourage disciplines of postgraduate study.

The editors said that Ralph E. Peterson, a Lutheran pastor, was the first president of the Minneapolis-based academy. Chapters would be organized throughout the country. In blocks of three years, members would be expected to complete 150 hours of continuing education divided between work performed in and work performed away from the parish. Members would spend half their time in nontheological areas of study. The editors closed by saying: "We salute the founders of the Academy of Parish Clergy and the vision with which they have given reality to a felicitous idea."

The Academy grew rapidly and soon included Roman Catholics and Jews. The academy still exists and is flourishing.[11]

Granger Is at It Again

While teaching at Hamma School of Theology, Granger was aware of the growing crisis in health care. The poor were not receiving adequate medical care. The number of general practitioners was dwindling. The cost of care was soaring. Middle-class families felt that they had less access to care. All of this propelled Granger forward in his conviction that the church should be more involved in helping people stay well. He had trained chaplains and provided courses for nurses. Professionally he had lived at the intersection of religion and medicine in major institutions. But what could local churches do? Granger had some ideas.

Chapter 15

Creating a Church Clinic

Although the US was one of the richest nations in the world, it had higher infant mortality rates and lower life expectancy rates than most European countries.[1] When Dwight L. Wilbur, president of the American Medical Association reported that 20 million people received inadequate medical care and called for ideas of ways to respond to the health care needs of all Americans, Granger was ready with ideas that he had been percolating for years. These ideas combined his interest in linking religion and medicine with a cost-effective strategy for providing care to the underserved. In a convocation address, he said:[2]

> We think the churches and synagogues of our land can make real contributions to the health of the nation. We propose an experimental program using certain church and synagogue buildings in inner city areas and in remote rural areas as neighborhood church-clinics. These would not simply be medical clinics that happen to be in churches and synagogues. They would constitute a new kind of relationship between medicine and religion.

Granger said thousands of churches and synagogues were virtually empty most of the week and that the clinics could be located in the education unit or other space. The churches could provide heat and light. The church clinics could offer more comprehensive care for the needs of the whole person. Qualified lay people could help in a variety of ways. For example, some could be trained as lay counselors who would be available to patients for listening and for conversation. In addition, church clinics could be excellent clinical teaching centers both for future ministers and future doctors. Granger said. "People in the neighborhood will find it easier to go to a nearby church clinic that is small, friendly, and inexpensive than to go to a distant hospital center that has the reputation of being overcrowded and impersonal and where the patient sees a different doctor on each visit."

Granger conceptualized the church clinic as "an action-research experiment to determine whether an ordinary congregation of people can assist physicians in providing health care to patients whose physical symptoms have been brought about chiefly by human problems, namely the stresses and strains of life."[3]

As a seminary professor who wanted his students to be able to relate theory to practice, Granger also saw a major role for his students in this experiment. Granger and some students from his practical theology class met with the principal, associate principal, and nurse from an elementary school located in a low-income neighborhood in Springfield, Ohio, where 15 percent of the people were unemployed. In this older neighborhood with narrow, crowded streets, about 80 percent of the people were Euro-Americans from Appalachia; 20 percent were African-Americans. After the visit, Granger, who had and would again receive good direction from nurses, wrote:

> She [the nurse] challenged us to take seriously that this was the sickest neighborhood in all of Springfield. She said that there were no physicians in the entire community; that when people were ill, they had to go to the hospital emergency room; and that the ambulance made more calls in this neighborhood than in any other neighborhood in Springfield.[4]

Fortuitously, Granger found a pastor in a neighborhood church, who was receptive to the idea of a church clinic project. The Rev. Jon Joyce had been pastor of Good Shepherd Church for two years. Although he and his parishioners (most of whom lived some distance from the neighborhood) were aware there were many needs in the neighborhood, they could not figure out how they could be of service.

Two seminarians experienced with sociological surveys created a survey designed to determine the areas of greatest need in the neighborhood and to ensure that the project would not duplicate existing governmental efforts. They also organized and trained a group of 10 seminarians to help interview members of the neighborhood on a random sample basis.

In visits to homes, the seminarians learned that there were no doctors' offices in the neighborhood and that it was very difficult for people in the neighborhood to get an appointment with a physician. Even local social workers reported calling as many as 18 physicians before they could find one who would accept a new patient.[5]

Local residents, schoolteachers, counselors, nurses, social workers, and clergy were enthusiastic about the proposed church clinic. Three community churches[6] agreed to join with Good Shepherd and co-sponsor the project.[7] Eventually the churches had representatives on the clinic's board of directors and members serving as volunteers in other capacities.

Granger presented the idea of the church clinic to the executive committee of the county medical society. Initially the members of the committee were opposed to the idea, saying there was no need for such a clinic in Springfield. Gradually, though, with further clarification from Granger, the physicians saw that the clinic would provide needed quality care and be a valid research project.[8]

Granger:

We could not have started our first church-clinic without the encouragement of Community Hospital. All of our planning—

which took nearly a year—was done in close collaboration with the hospital administrator and his staff as well as the members of the medical staff and the school of nursing faculty. The hospital supplied us with all the necessary equipment, such as used examining tables, autoclaves, and cabinets. Hospital personnel viewed the church clinic as a satellite clinic, helping to pick up the early cries for help from people who could be kept from getting sick enough to have to go to the hospital.

Three community physicians agreed to take turns volunteering their services on Wednesday afternoons. The list of nurses who volunteered to help was so long that not all of them were able to participate. In addition, arrangements were made for nursing students from Community Hospital's school of nursing to do some of their clinical training at the clinic.

Clergy from the sponsoring churches agreed to assist in providing counseling service. The Wheat Ridge Foundation and the Charles F. Kettering Foundation provided financial help. Lay people volunteered to greet patients, answer the phones, set up appointments, handle the finances, and babysit for children while parents were visiting with clinic staff members. Twenty volunteers from local churches were taught listening skills in a course called "How to Talk with People without Doing Too Much Harm."

The Church Clinic Opens

On February 4, 1970, with little fanfare apart from a door-to-door announcement to neighborhood households, the church clinic opened on a Wednesday afternoon-only basis. For that day and clinic days after that, the carpeted nursery became the exam room. Cribs and toys were put out of the way. In their place were small tables with tongue depressors, gauze, and scissors. White sheets were hung over wire for privacy. Sunday school rooms became counseling rooms.

Granger: "We were sure that a free clinic would attract more people than we would be able to handle, but it was weeks before the people in the neighborhood trusted us. Within three months, three to six people were being treated on an average afternoon. School nurses and social workers referred most of them. Seven months into the project, 20 to 30 patients were seen each Wednesday."

Later Granger and his colleagues learned that some neighborhood people had initially hesitated to come to the clinic because they were afraid that it was "some kind of gimmick that the churches were using it to get them to sit still to be preached at."[9]

One year after it opened, the church was swarming with people on clinic day. The available services had been expanded. In addition to the care provided by the physician and clergy, there was dental care, an eye clinic, and an immunization clinic with which public health nurses were involved. Counseling was provided on healthy lifestyles, marriage communication, and financial planning. There were courses on mothering, sewing, legal aid, and the care of cuts and burns. Student nurses worked under supervision.

Institutional medicine had shown interest in the project. The American Medical Association's Committee on Religion and Medicine, of which Granger was still a member, had approved the clinic as a pilot project. The National Institutes of Health and several medical school deans requested progress reports.[10]

In the early 1970s it was assumed that only liberal congregations would be involved in social action. Granger challenged that notion:[11]

The Good Shepherd Church is a typical conservative congregation made up of middle class people who have never done anything more risky than have a day care center for children. To date we have received wholehearted cooperation from all members of the congregation because they see a church clinic as being in line with Christ's command to go preach and heal. Even the church sexton goes the extra mile in cleaning up after the clinic because he feels that he is involved in a meaningful ministry to people who are hurting. He participates from time to time in discussions with patients, and has found new meaning in his ministry.

Funds from the Kettering Foundation of Dayton made it possible for Dr. Karl Hertz, a clergy-sociologist, who taught both at Wittenberg University and Hamma School of Theology, to work with some of his graduate students in studying the project. A year after the clinic was open, Hertz and his team did in-depth interviews of a random sampling of the 225 families who were receiving their health care at the clinic.[12] Prior to going to the church clinic, many respondents said they had been having difficulty getting health care. Some resisted going to hospital clinics "because of what they may do to you." In contrast, at the church clinic, "They ask you what you think. They don't just go over your head or tell you to shut up." Generally patients felt that the church clinic physicians were "more intent on finding your illness," "more thorough," and spent "more time with you." than physicians at other facilities.

Most people felt very positive about ministers helping people when they were ill. Responses included: "Illness comes different ways. It helps to talk to a minister about how it got started. Then he can better tell the doctor." "If you feeling like givin' up, then medicine will do you no good. But the minister can talk to you and show you that everything is still worth you still tryin' and goin' on and livin.'"

A year and a half after the church clinic opened, Don Tubesing, a young minister who had heard Granger talking about the clinic six months earlier at a meeting of Ohio clergy, paid a visit. Don had been intrigued by what Granger said and regarded Granger as a "prophet in the wilderness." He was eager to learn more about the church clinic. Don reflected:[13]

On the day I visited the clinic, the clinic appeared much as I had expected—an old church in an old neighborhood ... Certainly an unlikely place for a revolution. There were three or four people in the waiting room near the basement entrance. Mr. Miller, a regular volunteer trouble-shooter was there. A couple of other people were walking around. There was nothing special at all ... at first glance. A tour, however, revealed a mother and daughter finding some "new" clothes in the sewing and exchange room at the end of the hall, a young seminarian introducing two neighbors to each other in the waiting room, and Granger teaching a class of student nurses on wholistic medicine in the chapel upstairs.

The nursery was being used as an exam room. A dental chair was in the ladies' choir room. The men's choir room and some Sunday school rooms were busy with counseling sessions.

All over the church, quietly, almost unnoticed, 10 to 12 volunteer doctors, ministers, nurses, and lay people were busy meeting with patients and responding to their health care needs. Nothing was rigid or formal—sweaters not ties, slacks not uniforms were the attire. Warmth, patience, and an attitude of 'taking the time' were evident.

Was the project as impressive as I had hoped? Well, yes and no! To my normal way of viewing, it wasn't impressive at all—just simple folk in a simple building doing simple easygoing things. But it was more than could be viewed with the naked eye. Seen through the eye of human concern and the vision of the potential embodied in the efforts of that place, it was quite impressive indeed.

There was a great deal of public interest in the clinic. Articles appeared in newspapers. A crew from NBC spent several days at the clinic and produced a piece on the church clinic that was aired nationally. Shortly after Don Tubesing's visit, a reporter from *The National Observer* visited the clinic and wrote:[14]

> I came to Springfield as a skeptic about this new approach to medical care. Tell it to the chaplain—ha! I left, however, convinced that the church clinic functions effectively.
>
> ... Today's materialistic people, I thought, sure wouldn't be so old-fashioned as to spill their woes to a minister, especially one "out of place" in a medical clinic. I was wrong. The patients ache, worry, and need help, and if a clergyman can provide it, fine. Besides, these clergymen are low-keyed and unpretentious. They conscientiously assist a patient no matter what his religious belief or lack of it."

After two years the clinic hours were expanded to four and one-half days each week. The large number of patients who came to the clinic, the positive feedback given by patients on surveys, and the decreasing use of area emergency vehicles by neighborhood residents were indicators that the clinic was responding successfully to a human need by providing low cost but sound medical care, which focused on the whole person.[15] The many volunteers were helpful.

Volunteers at the front desk in the clinic reported that some of the men who initially resisted seeing a minister on their first visit returned a second time. One man indicated that he had appreciated the last visit with the minister because it was the first time that he felt someone had really listened to him. A volunteer reported that one man, who came back for a second visit, leaned over the desk and in a quiet voice said, "I'm not sure that I need to see a doctor, but I would like to talk to one of the ministers."[16]

Granger:[17] It took a while for people to understand why a minister would be interested in problems of health care. But when they found that we were not in a hurry and were willing to help them ventilate their true feelings, the patients themselves often mentioned the close relation between their inner spirit and their health."

Contextual Teaching of Pastoral Care

Granger reflected on the benefits of the church clinic project for him and his teaching:[18]

> Perhaps the chief value of this project is that I have been forced to do more and more of my teaching outside the seminary walls. I am increasingly convinced that it would probably be better if almost all pastoral care and counseling were taught on location where the people are.
>
> ... We do not need artificial props, role-playing or statements of "how to do it when you get out." The students are there! This is not a theory course. Students are ministering to real people with real problems and then reflecting on what they have done, why they have done it in a particular way, how their style of ministry can be improved, and how what they are doing is related to what they believe about the nature of God and God's good news.

Since he began teaching in the church clinic, Granger said that he was increasingly aware of how "unreal" the atmosphere was in seminary classrooms where everything was "sterile" and "orderly," and there were no interruptions of the professor's teaching. "Our teaching at the church," he said, "is constantly interrupted by real life situations. At first that was terribly frustrating, but then we realized that it is only as the student actually participates in ministry and then is forced to reflect deeply on what he is doing, that quality learning takes place."

Granger and his students saw patients together. Often he observed in the background while a student interviewed a patient. Sometimes the student watched Granger interview patients. Occasionally Granger and a student jointly interviewed a patient. Following the patient visit, Granger and the student reflected on the visit, by themselves or with others in something of an instant seminar.[19]

Doctors, nurses, and lay people also taught the seminarians informally, but occasionally they joined in impromptu seminars at the clinic. Granger said that many times the lay people's suggestions were the most practical and helpful.

In addition to meeting with students on the day of the clinic, Granger met with them for three hours on another day. The students took turns presenting written case studies and then reflected together on the theological and other dimensions of the patients' situations.

About a year and a half after the neighborhood clinic was underway, Granger was invited to speak at Howard Medical School in Washington DC. There, members of the primarily African-American audience presented a challenge that was to change the direction of the project. Granger recalled:

> They said, "We like your idea. To deal with the spiritual dimension of people and to work with people in Act 1 is very important. But are you only going to do this in poor neighborhoods?" I replied that, yes, that's all I had really thought about. "Well," they said, "if you put it only in low-income neighborhoods, you're going to give the impression that this is just poor people's medicine. If these poor people ever get money, they won't want that kind of medicine. They'll want what the rich people have—pure scientific medicine without any of this counseling and health education business."
>
> Someone else continued, "Why don't you start a clinic in a middle-class neighborhood church where people can afford to pay their way? You could pay the doctor, a nurse and a pastor a fair wage and make it pay for itself." Another student added, "Why don't you even do it in a rich neighborhood? Those people need it more than anybody!"

Granger reflected a great deal on these challenges from the students at Howard. In time, he accepted their challenge.

To create other church clinics, Granger needed funding. One of the foundations he approached was the W. K. Kellogg Foundation. The Kellogg staff had some interest in Granger's work, so they sent Robert DeVries, a staff member, to Springfield to meet with Granger and others. Granger was pleased that Bob was coming. As a student in hospital administration at the University of Chicago, Bob had been one of Granger's students. Bob and Granger also shared things Lutheran, as Bob had been president of Lutheran Student Parish at the university. Bob also had experience in health care in Ohio. He had spent eight years at Miami Valley Hospital in Dayton, where, as assistant director, the chaplaincy department was one of his responsibilities.

Hotel accommodations in Springfield were minimal, so Bob stayed overnight with Helen, Granger, and Jill. The next morning Bob was wakened to the sound of hymns being played on an organ. When he came downstairs, Granger was playing "Now Thank We All Our God" on a pump organ. Subsequently, in a few public speeches, Bob talked about waking up to Granger's music at the Westberg house.

In anticipation of Bob's visit, Helen had bought several Kellogg breakfast cereals. Helen: "In the morning when I asked Bob what he would like to eat, he said, 'Bacon and eggs.'"

Always Finding the Bright Side

Hamma, like more than 10 other theological seminaries in the Lutheran Church in America, was in financial trouble. The church-at-large wanted Hamma and the other seminaries to merge, so there would be fewer seminaries. Granger: "Our faculty met a number of times with the faculty from the seminary with which we were to merge [Trinity Lutheran Theological Seminary in Columbus, Ohio]. It was clear that the faculty from the other seminary was quite conservative and that there would not be many opportunities to try new things."

At the end of the school year, Granger would be without a salary and without a base, but, as was so often the case, he saw the bright side: "The merger came at just the right time for me because I was dreaming about starting four neighborhood church clinics: one in an upper-income neighborhood, one in a middle-income neighborhood, a third in a very low-income neighborhood, and one in a rural church. With all my contacts in the Chicago area and with all its churches, synagogues, theological schools, hospitals, and medical schools, I thought Chicago would be a good place to search for the kind of support I needed."

Later, reflecting on this period in their life, Helen, who often had to be the realist in order to balance Granger's tendency to be inordinately optimistic, said, "Granger was excited about his dream. I had the more practical slant on it."

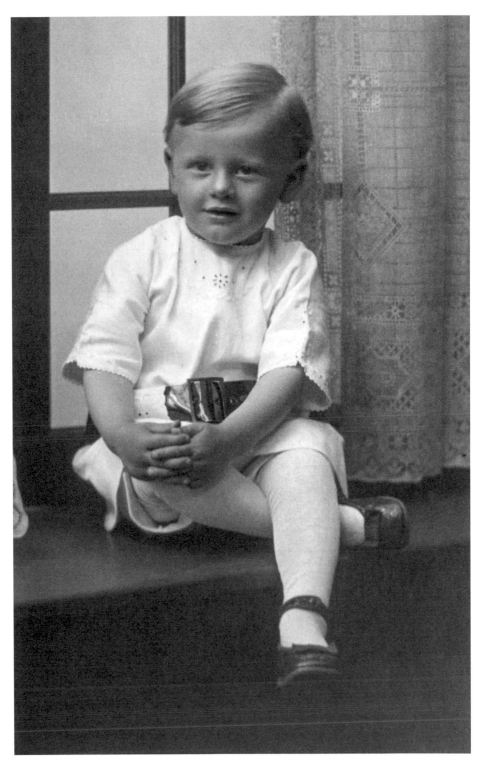

Granger, age 2.

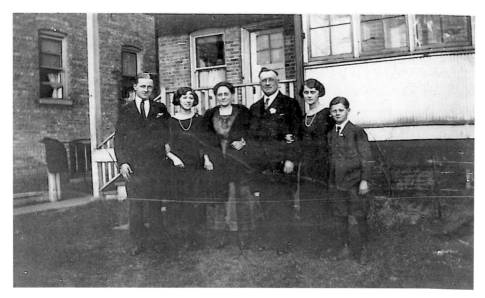

John and Alma (Ahlstrom) Westberg's 25th wedding anniversary, 1923. Orville, Eulalia, Alma, John, Viola and Granger.

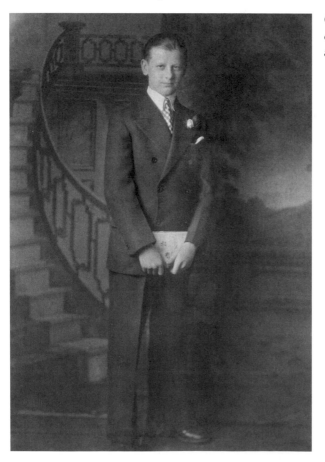

Granger's confirmation, age 14.

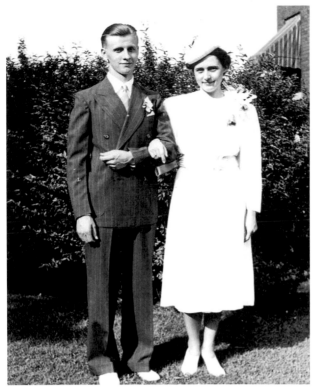

After putting himself through school during the Depression, Granger weighed the same as or less than Helen Johnson on their wedding day, 1939.

Granger and Helen with Jane, age 1, in 1942.

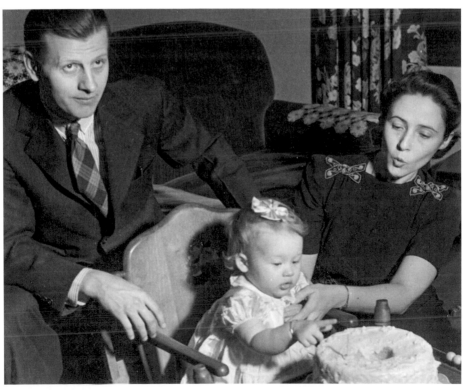

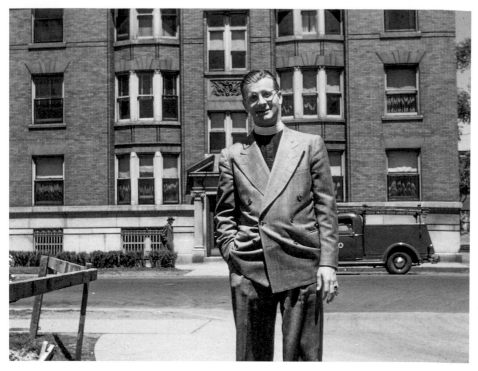

Chaplain Granger Westberg in front of Augustana Hospital.

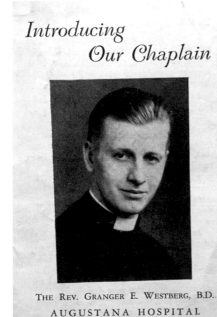

Introducing
Our Chaplain

THE REV. GRANGER E. WESTBERG, B.D.
AUGUSTANA HOSPITAL
(Lutheran)
CHICAGO, ILLINOIS

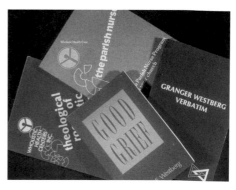

Granger was a prolific writer of articles and books. *Good Grief*, published in 1962, became a best seller.

When Granger became chaplain of Augustana Hospital in 1944, he was one of the early clinically educated Protestant chaplains.

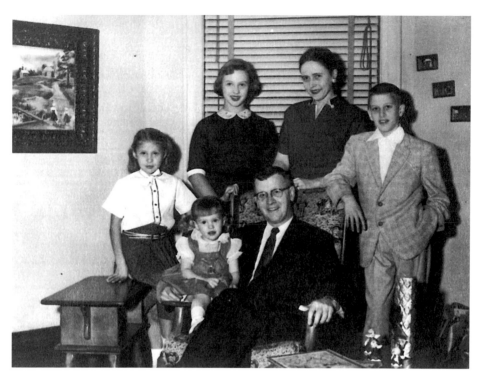

Westberg family Christmas photo, 1956. Joan, Jane, Helen, John, Jill and Granger.

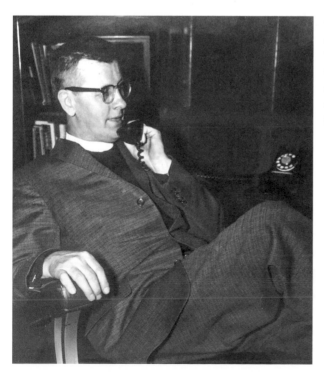

Granger at his University of Chicago office, around 1956, after receiving the first known joint appointment in schools of divinity and medicine at a major university.

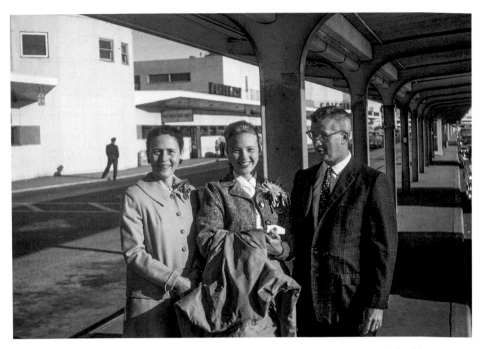

Helen and Granger see Jane off in 1959 for her flight to the UK to attend the University of Edinburgh.

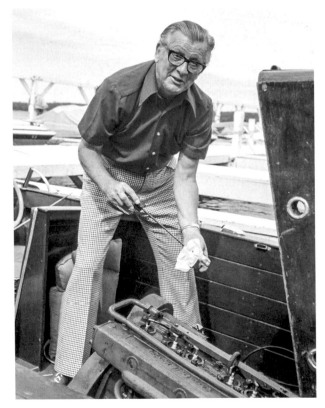

Known for gently rocking the boat in his profession, Granger also enjoyed working on and giving friends rides in his boat on Lake Geneva, near the beloved, longtime family cabin, 1979.

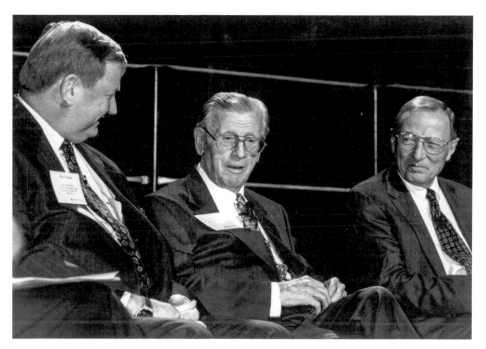

Robert Baylor, Granger Westberg and George Caldwell at the 1996 Westberg Symposium. Baylor was head of the spiritual care work at Evangelical Health System. Caldwell was president of Lutheran General Health System and a generous supporter of Westberg.

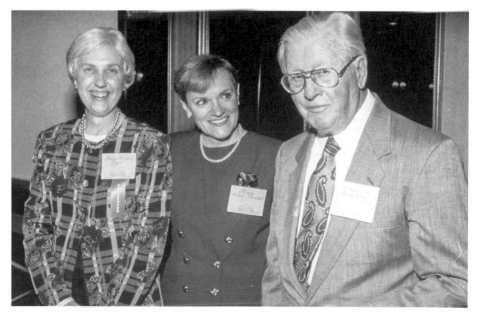

Anne Marie Djupe, Ann Solari-Twadell, and Granger at a 1990s Westberg Symposium. Djupe and Solari-Twadell, both nurses, helped create and launch the parish nurse movement, later known as faith community nursing.

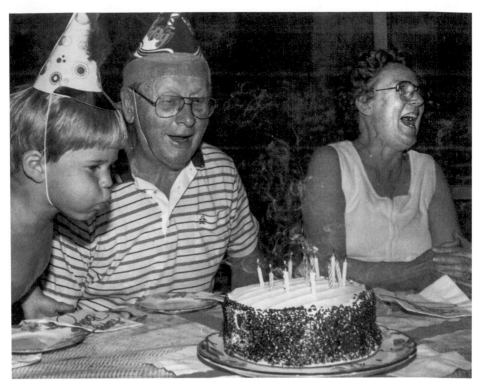

Granger's birthday in 1988. Grandson Ian (Jill's son) helps him blow out his candles. Helen enjoys the fun.

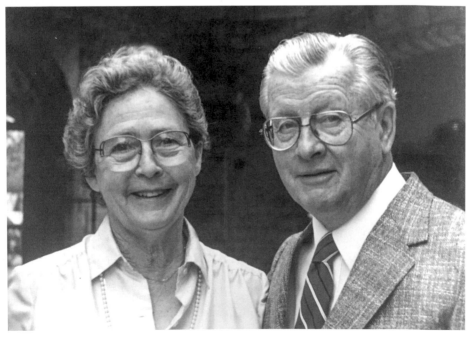

Helen and Granger in the 1980s.

Chapter 16

A 30-Year Dream

The church clinic in Springfield, Ohio, was doing well, but was its success due to the fact that it was located in a medically underserved neighborhood and the care was free? Granger was eager to test whether such clinics (or "Wholistic Health Centers" as he was now beginning to call them) could be successful in churches and synagogues in middle and upper-income communities.

Early in 1972, before moving from Springfield, Ohio, back to the Chicago area, Granger began searching Chicago for support for creating a church clinic in a middle- or upper-income community. For months he had meetings with clergy, seminary professors, medical educators, nursing educators, hospital administrators, and foundations. At each meeting he told the story of the Springfield clinic and his dreams of Wholistic Health Centers. Administrators of several theological schools agreed to place students at the Wholistic Health Centers but said they couldn't fund the centers. Then, following the advice of a potential funding agency, Granger focused on finding a medical school that had a department of community and preventive medicine, a department of family medicine, or both. Since the University of Chicago had neither, he had to look elsewhere.

When Granger spoke directly with administrators and educators at the medical schools, he often got them excited about his dream. But then the bureaucracy or the skepticism of others in the school squelched plans for action. Also, some of the key people Granger was trying to reach were on vacation, interim assignments, or leaves of absence.

The dean of Northwestern University School of Medicine in Evanston, Illinois, was open to testing Granger's dream. However, he said that the project would be in the province of the new chair of preventive medicine, so they would have to wait until this physician arrived.

Writing to the Rev. Dean F. Lueking, pastor of a large Lutheran church in a Chicago suburb, Granger said: "I have decided to take the leap of faith and give myself full time to develop my 30-year dream to bring ministers and doctors together in caring for the whole patient." As Granger later said, "I was convinced that I was on the right track."

Helen: "But we took a gamble. We were without a job and living on savings. We left Springfield in June, not knowing where we were going to move. We took our personal things up to Lake Geneva, where we planned to live for the summer, and left the rest of our belongings in Springfield. On one of his visits to Evanston, Granger found a house and bought it without asking me first. (This was the only time he did that.) The yard of the Evanston house was very beautiful. The house left a lot to be desired."

Shortly after Helen and Granger were beginning to feel settled in their new home in Evanston, the new chair of preventive medicine, a surgeon, arrived at Northwestern. As a physician oriented to treating disease, he did not see the merit in Granger's project.

A friend suggested that Granger contact Edward Lichter, the new chair of the department of preventive medicine and community health of the Abraham Lincoln School of Medicine at University of Illinois in Chicago. Granger:

My friend said that Lichter was a very good man, but he said, "You probably wouldn't be interested because he's Jewish." I said, "On the contrary. I've found that more Jewish doctors are interested in what we're doing than Christian doctors."

When I met Lichter I told him about what we had already done with the church clinic in Springfield and how medical students at Howard had challenged us to try the model out in a variety of neighborhoods. He seemed interested, so I continued.

When I finished, he said, "I think what you're planning is very sound, both medically and theologically." Taken aback, I said, "Oh, I didn't expect to hear you use the word *theological*. He said, "Well after all, this whole business of wholistic medicine is really what your man Jesus did." Then he caught himself and said, "I mean our man Jesus." He continued, "The problem is, you Christians got screwed up by those Greeks who divided man into two parts: body and soul. They've given the body to us doctors and the souls to you ministers, and we haven't talked with each other in 2,000 years."

We talked and talked. I submitted a proposal to him, and soon he arranged for me to have a faculty appointment. We were off and running. It was the beginning of a wonderful relationship."

Granger talked with Ed Lichter about turning to the Kellogg Foundation for support, explaining he already had met with Bob DeVries, a program director with Kellogg. Ed wrote the Kellogg Foundation an enthusiastic letter of support for Granger's proposal. Soon arrangements were made for Granger to talk again with Bob DeVries.

Granger said, "After hearing my story, Bob asked, 'What do you think you need in the way of money?' As I talked through what I thought the expenses would be, he wrote them down on a chalkboard. When I finished, the total came to $75,000. Bob said, 'I just don't think we can do that.' Very disappointed, I asked, 'What do you mean?' Bob said, 'We've got to do this thing right or not at all.'" This wonderful advisor was conveying the message that it would take, and that they would provide, more money to do the project properly.

In April 1973, the Kellogg Foundation provided generous funding for a four-year grant to the University of Illinois with Dr. Ed Lichter as the principal investigator. Ed brought Granger into his department as a full-time faculty member.

The First Wholistic Health Center Home

For the first Wholistic Health Center (WHC), Granger needed a church with a supportive staff and adequate facilities and resources. He wanted the church to be located in a middle-income community with many doctors, a good local hospital, and a medically sophisticated population. He also wanted the church to be within reasonable driving distance of teaching hospitals and seminaries.

The pastor of the Lutheran church in La Grange in which Granger and family had been members considered the proposal but did not think that he or the congregation were ready for it. However, Sidney Lovett, pastor of Union Church (United Church of Christ), in Hinsdale, an affluent western suburb of Chicago, was interested. Within two weeks of speaking to Granger, he secured his congregation's agreement to put a Wholistic Health Center in their church.

Granger:

People in Hinsdale asked, "Why are you thinking of starting a Center in Hinsdale where we've got more doctors than we need?" My reply was that I had to test this model in the midst of the finest medical care obtainable, with people who could afford to pay for anything they needed. If I could show that people would come to a doctor's office in a church and see others for help, such as a pastor well-trained in counseling and a nurse well-trained in health education, preventive medicine, and nutrition; and if we could supplement this with regular educational courses, seminars, and workshops; if we can prove that this type of care is desired in Hinsdale, people would come to a Center any place.

Granger and Helen also found a home in the suburb of Downers Grove, a short drive from the Hinsdale church. Jill lived close by in a George Williams College dorm. John lived 20 minutes away with his wife and two-year-old son, Jimmy.

Getting Started

Ever since Don Tubesing heard Granger speak in Ohio and then visited the church clinic in Springfield, he kept in touch with Granger. Don, who had both a master's of divinity degree and a doctorate in counseling, had recently moved from Ohio to Wisconsin, where he was dean of student affairs at a small college. The day after the Kellogg grant was awarded, Granger offered Donald Tubesing the position of associate director. Later Don wrote:[1]

> I picked up the phone a number of times to tell Granger, "No, I'm not coming." But I'd never been able to actually call and say it. Something lured me. It was July 1, 1973 when I first arrived for work, ready to dig in. I remember the place needed sprucing up. Would wealthy people used to first-rate technical care in well-decorated offices come to this church basement for medical care? I must admit, sorry to say, I had my doubts.
>
> My most impressive memory of that day was that nothing was happening. Almost no one was there, just Granger, Paul Holinger (a medical student on a clerkship) and me. Granger had an office, but there were no patients, no furniture, no staff, no procedures, just a vision. "Well friends, what shall we do today? Where shall we start?" was the way Granger got the day rolling.

Gradually the church basement started looking like a clinic. An examination table arrived, along with other medical furniture and equipment. Nurses and clergy with education in counseling applied for positions. Others volunteered.

In September 1973 the Center was given a boost by a health-screening program that was held at the Center and cosponsored by the Hinsdale Sanitarium and Hospital. Roughly 1,300 persons came through the clinic in four days of testing and health education. The staff also spread the word about the Center by giving 100 courses, lectures, seminars, and sermons in local churches during that first year, often to groups of 100–300 people. However, Granger wrote:[2]

> Our suburban audience was more difficult to convince of the validity of our approach than was the low-income neighborhood clientele in Springfield, Ohio. Even though the suburban people responded enthusiastically to every presentation, they always thought of the Wholistic Health Centers as something that was good for someone else they knew. They were not quite ready to see themselves needing an approach that dealt with the need to look at how their lifestyle might be contributing to illness.

Eventually, people did start coming. A few were even referred by local physicians.

By October 1973, the volunteer staff included three pastoral counselors, three nurses, two secretary receptionists, and a director of volunteer services. The recruitment of physicians, however, was another matter. Local physicians could not be enticed to volunteer as they had done in Springfield. Most had very active full-time practices. Finally, two physicians who had young children and only wanted to work part-time signed on.

Volunteers served in every phase of the life of the Center. In addition to the health professionals who gave their professional services, some volunteers served as members of the advisory committee. Others helped with day-to-day administrative and secretarial tasks. Still others worked directly with patients—making introductions, answering questions, serving coffee, and in general creating a friendly supportive anxiety-reducing atmosphere.

Nurses at the Hub of Care

The style of patient care in the WHC was similar to that of the church clinic in Springfield, except, as Don noted, the role of the nurse was dramatically changed to that of "patient advocate":[3]

> The nurse, rather than the pastor, became the key coordinator of a patient's visit. She made certain that the patient knew ahead of time what to expect and received the kind of help he or she was seeking. Whenever appropriate, the nurse stayed with the patient throughout the visit, introduced the patient to the other professional staff members, and helped make arrangements for necessary tests and the scheduling of return visits. She often asked for feedback: "Did you get the kind of help you wanted? What would you like to see happen as we proceed?" As much as possible, the same nurse was assigned to the patient on each return visit.

People who came to the WHC could receive straightforward help from the nurse or the doctor for their complaint, but they also were given the option of having an Initial Health Planning Conference. This conference began with patients filling out a personal health inventory that included questions about the patient's complaint and past illnesses and surgeries. The inventory also included questions about the patient's strengths and support systems and questions about recent life events that can affect health, such as divorce and children going off to college.

After completing the inventory, the patient met with a health team comprised of the physician, nurse, and pastor. The patient was a key member of the team. Using the inventory as one of the tools for the discussion, the patient and the team not only addressed the patient's immediate concerns but also began developing long-term goals and strategies for achieving these goals.

At the close of each clinic day, the entire staff gathered for a conference. They discussed patient needs and identified and worked at solving problems. An important task was reflecting on whether their work was embodying the center's wholistic philosophy and, if not, what they could do to ensure that their values and work were in alignment.

Granger and his colleagues continued to struggle with how to make the Wholistic Health Center work in an affluent neighborhood. Don:[4] "Whereas in Springfield, Ohio, the counseling aspect of the clinic needed to be emphasized so that it didn't get lost, in Hinsdale, the opposite seemed true. The pastoral counseling image was heard and accepted; it was the medical that got lost." The Springfield model could not be simply transported. For the Center to attract more than a handful of local people, it had to be fully comparable on a medical basis with other medical clinics in the area.

So the staff went to work. The facilities were remodeled in order to add a "stainless steel medical look" to the clinic. Two important changes in the second year were the addition of a physician who had recently returned from a medical mission in Liberia and the opening of a second WHC. Granger and his colleagues wanted to test the WHC in another setting.

Chapter 17

As a Matter of Faith

Don Tubesing became the pastoral director of the second WHC located in the Woodridge United Methodist Church. Woodridge was a new middle-class Chicago suburb with a highly mobile population and a lack of medical services. William Peterson, an ordained minister in the United Church of Christ with master's degrees both in theology and social work, took Don's position as pastoral director at Hinsdale.

Don and his skeleton staff spent the first few months gathering and training staff, including a full-time nurse, four volunteer nurses, and five volunteer ministers from the community. The next three months, with the help of 100 community volunteers, the Center held 10 luncheons for local ministers, teachers, principals, counselors, physicians and social workers during which the staff told their story and got acquainted with the local leaders. In addition, close to 100 people attended a six-week creative management of stress course run by the staff. Further, over 600 people attended a health fair at the Center.

As a result of these activities, Don wrote:[1] "... not only did the patient load increase, but just as importantly, the community people began to feel a sense of ownership and pride in 'their' Wholistic Health Center. It was no longer just a few staff people from the University of Illinois at the Medical Center in Chicago doing 'their thing' in Woodridge. Volunteers, church and community people were actively involved in planning and making decisions as to the future Wholistic Health Center Programs."

Writing in retrospect about the end of the second year of the project, Don reported that the health education efforts at both centers expanded steadily and now included courses and groups focusing on smoking cessation, marriage, family planning, parent-teenage communication, self-care, grief, and aging. In many of these sessions, the participants drew on their own experiences and learning and were able to teach each other.

Both WHCs were moving toward being self-supporting, but, as evidenced by this December 1974 memo from Ed Lichter, there was a ways to go. "Dear Granger: Just a reminder that you are now averaging a project annual income of $12–13,000. You'll have to triple that just to meet expenses. Have you thought of selling apples? Ed."

On October 24, 1975, in an article in the *Washington Star*, reporter Christine Russell, who was aware of the "holistic" health care activities on the west coast as well as the efforts of Granger and his colleagues, wrote:

> In contrast to many West Coast-based efforts, Westberg's WHCs are designed to appeal to the more conventionally-minded patient who's nevertheless been turned off by the present health care system. An experimental program he started in Hinsdale three years ago seems to be prospering because it provides an old-fashioned blend of traditional medicine and personal consultation, which few customers can find elsewhere.
>
> Westberg's centers strive instead to work within the establishment, even down to the physical setup. After first making the clinics look informal, he now encourages the "doctor to wear doctors' clothes and the nurse smocks."

During the third year of the project, (1975–1976), health promotion-disease-preventive programs were expanded as were patient education seminars. Scores of courses were offered. A new addition was the annual employees health evaluation program conducted for businesses. This was a two-stage process, including a full physical examination and a personal lifestyle assessment.

Rocking the Boat Gently

Robert M. Cunningham, Jr., a member of the staff of the national Blue Cross Association and contributing editor to *Modern Healthcare*, did a thorough study of the Wholistic Health Centers, for the W. K. Kellogg Foundation. In his foreword to Cunningham's resulting monograph, Walter J. McNerney, president of Blue Cross, wrote that along with others who also were involved in financing the delivery of health services, he was convinced that "a larger share of our resources should be directed toward teaching and motivating people to be healthy." He referred to the WHC as a "promising activity" and praised its creative use of church facilities and services. "I am encouraging Blue Cross Plans to help the wholistic centers that are getting started ... in every way they can, just as I have encouraged them to take part in preventive medicine and health education programs of all kinds for the last several years. In the absence of outcome data, I am convinced as a matter of faith that wholistic care makes sense; it is an intelligent adaptation to the complex conditions of the post communicable disease era."

In preparing for writing his "experience report" for Kellogg, Cunningham had visited both Wholistic Health Centers, interviewed the staff and others, attended talks given by Granger and others, and engaged in additional information-gathering activities. His summary, which also refers to the clinic in Springfield, included the following:[2]

> After six years of trial, there is a possibility, at least, that Granger
> Westberg's vision that the under-used resources of American
> churches and America's clergy may be set in motion to improve
> America's health, will be realized. If this should happen, it will

certainly be because of Dr. Westberg's dedicated efforts over the years and because of the energy and enthusiasm of those who have been willing to leave secure professional careers to become associated with the Wholistic Health Centers ... But it will also be because the concept is in consonance with a new mode of thought that has been emerging in recent years among leaders of medicine and the other health professions, a movement that has been referred to variously as "the new medicine," and "humanistic medicine," and "(w)holistic medicine."

The report gave Granger and his colleagues encouragement that they were moving in the right direction.

In the third annual report to the Kellogg Foundation, Granger noted a shift in local physicians' reaction to the Centers: "The survey of some 300 physicians in the area got an unusually high rate of response, namely 59%. We were surprised and pleased to learn how many physicians had recommended the clinics to their patients, one physician recommending them to 30 patients. In other words ... we pose less of a threat to doctors and are seen as a resource for certain patients."

Writing about the WHCs in *Medical Care*, Don Tubesing, Paul Holinger, Granger, and Edward Lichter[3] titled their article: "The Wholistic Health Center Project: An Action-research Model for Providing Preventive, Whole-Person Health Care at the Primary Level." They noted that one of the many positive features of the Wholistic Health Centers was the fact that the centers provided "an entry into the health care system for persons who 'just aren't feeling well' but do not yet feel they are sick and, therefore, would not seek regular medical care." They also wrote that one of the stated goals of the project was "to mobilize the multitude of people-helping-people resources within the local church communities and bring them to bear on individual and community health problems." Patients were being put into contact with other people who had similar health difficulties and had learned to cope creatively.

Responding to concerns by some people about whether proselytizing was occurring at the WHCs, the authors responded that clergy counselors were not interested in proselytizing. Rather, as "an expert in the faith/value dimension of human life," the counselor "helps the patient sort out the meanings in his/her life and identify the value conflicts that may be contributing to stress and illness." In addition to typical counseling approaches, the pastoral counselor might also ask such questions as "What is the aim of your life?" "What beliefs and values guide you?" and "What are you willing to let go of?" Patients often respond to these challenges, the authors said, "by exploring their lifestyles and making appropriate health-related behavioral changes."

The WHC model was being tested in an affluent community (Hinsdale) and in a highly mobile middle class community (Woodridge). Granger and his supporters also wanted to test the WHC model in other settings. In 1976 a WHC was opened in a rural community in Mendota, Illinois, 70 miles west of Chicago. Great community spirit and a sense of ownership was engendered when the people in Mendota raised close to $19,000 to remodel the church that was to be used as a clinic. This caused the WHC staff to feel that people at all new WHCs should be asked to raise some of their own funds. The Mendota WHC was given a big jumpstart when Dr. Lucy Young became medical director and moved her practice of 2,000 patients into the church center.

The Austin-Chicago WHC, later called "Circle Wholistic Health Center," was opened in 1977 in a low-income largely African-American community in Chicago. The WHC was set up by a group that included physicians, nurses, an attorney and at least one pastor who had been students together at the Circle Campus of the University of Illinois in Chicago. In the same building, patients had access to legal aid, homemakers' services, and a practical learning center for youth.

In an April 3, 1977 article in the *Chicago Sun Times* reporter Allan Parachini described his visit with Granger:

> Mr. Westberg's office in the Union Church has become the center of national attention for his notion that churches have not only the space but a unique atmosphere for getting people to think of health in terms broader than the absence of sickness. As he talked about his work last week, organ music was heard from the main wing of the church. The organist was practicing for the Sunday service. "Church buildings are delightful places," Granger said, "What doctor's office has music like this? This is a happy place … a healthy place. Why not put health care in a healthy place?"

Parachini noted that until recently the Wholistic Health Center projects had gotten only a modest amount of publicity. He continued:

> But then in February, Mr. Westberg flew to New York for a brief appearance at a conference of health policy makers. The conference was intended to plan for a revolution in health concepts for health care delivery. This panel, attended by just 8 people, was one of the smallest on the program. But John Knowles, President of the Rockefeller Foundation, wandered into the room and was struck by the simplicity of what Mr. Westberg was saying. Mr. Westberg became a conference celebrity.

Parachini reported that Granger was "rocking the boat gently." He added that since the conference Granger had more than 25 serious inquiries about the WHCs.

A National Office

Within the first few years of the WHC project, 300 people from

Seattle to Boston visited the WHC with a view to starting a WHC in their communities. Several of the groups included administrators and physicians who represented hospitals. This growing interest in the Wholistic Health Centers made it clear that it was time to create a national office to assist such groups in planning and developing WHCs.

In 1976, with funding from W. K. Kellogg, the national office called "Wholistic Health Centers, Inc." was established with the goal of providing leadership to the Wholistic Health Center movement and handling the administrative responsibilities for the Wholistic Health Centers projects. Granger was president of Wholistic Health Centers, Inc; Don Tubesing was vice president and director of programs. Kent Savage, a longtime board member, and others served as consultants for the business aspects of the national office. Community leaders, including clergy and physicians, provided additional help.

In 1977, John Riedel, who had a master's degree in public health, joined the national office as director of clinical development. John remembered that joining the national office was like joining a family: "Granger didn't make an offer to me until he had met with my wife, Mary. He wanted to make sure that this was something she wanted too. She came away from that meeting very committed, happy, and pleased."

Early in 1977 Granger's youngest daughter, Jill, joined the staff of Wholistic Health Centers Inc. on a part-time basis while she finished college. Jill remembered,

> In all honesty, Dad's invitation to hire me was an effort to help me choose a "suitable" career. My winter job consisted of teaching a few classes of therapeutic horseback riding, but most of my time was spent shoveling manure. Somehow Dad didn't see that as the best plan for advancement. He hired me feeling sure, as always, that the best careers were in religion or health, preferably both.

I was leery about working with Dad, especially since through my teenage years he and I, like many other parents and teens, had our differences. But the novelty of shoveling manure during a Chicago winter had worn off and so I accepted his offer. Working at WHC, Inc. put me in a position that was all about change. In our work together Dad and I were both finally headed in the same direction.

I was living at home so Dad and I talked faith and health over dinner and on our commute to and from work. He included me in meetings, giving me a sense of future possibilities and decisions being made. One of the last courses I took in college was an independent study on "hope." Dad and my boss, Bill Peterson, liked the paper and included it in a WHC monograph.[4] Pretty soon I was helping to write our newsletter, planning the national staff conferences and helping with the organization of the upcoming national symposium. Watching Dad interact with other professionals and seeing how much respect he had for each person and their thoughts, my admiration for him grew.

Chapter 18

Life Is a Leaky Boat

One of the highlights of 1977 was the National Invitational Symposium on Wholistic Health Care. It brought together national level leaders in health care policy, theological education, medical education, nursing education, government, the consumer movement, and private industry. Five people from Kellogg were there.

Russell Mawby, president of the W. K. Kellogg Foundation, told the group that Kellogg saw the project "as a model that takes into account the whole person, that provides personalized care, that is comprehensive in nature, that embraces the notions of self-responsibility, health promotion, and health education and emphasizes preventive medicine ... We have been following with special interest the experiences of this project."

Bernard Siegel, dean of the School of Medicine at the University of Illinois, said he was interested in the project because his university wanted to "help develop new and innovative approaches to health care." Also, he said, "We are interested in finding an appropriate model for the teaching of preventive medicine and health."

Granger described the three acts of illness and the need to put more resources into Act 1:

Public health nurses, counselors, teachers, and clergy focus on health care rather than sickness care. Both the clergy and schoolteachers get to know whole families and maintain the acquaintance over a period of time ... They are in touch with the stresses of life, which contribute greatly to the onset of illness in its earliest stages. Their knowledge needs to be tapped and taken seriously in the health care system.

I have yet to hear a physician react with anything but surprise when I ask whether he has thought of involving the minister. But involve him we must. It is not necessary for a huge percentage of physicians to suddenly start working in Act 1. This involvement would not efficiently use their high level of technical training. It is necessary, however, to take seriously the educators, clergy, counselors, nurse practitioners, and others with expertise and interest in the preventive efforts necessary for assisting persons in the first Act of Illness—before they get sicker.

Walter J. McNerney, president of Blue Cross Blue Shield, enumerated the obstacles facing Wholistic Health Centers:

1. Cultural disposition of physicians and hospitals to be concerned with sickness, not health.
2. Understandable reluctance of physicians to acknowledge any need for the assistance of non-physicians in the diagnosis and treatment of illness.
3. Third party payment for the services the Centers are providing.

McNerney said he didn't know how long it would take for public policy to "catch on to the fact that apprehension may be as treatable an illness as appendicitis." Meanwhile, he said, "I can assure you that I shall do all I can to urge Blue Cross and Blue Shield Plans and other payers to accept the ultimate economy of a healthier population and work in their communities to encourage the development of wholistic centers, including payment for the widest possible range of services provided by the centers."

Theologian Joseph Sittler, Granger's colleague and friend of many decades, noted: "What's happening in the conversation we're having is happening all over the culture. For about 400 years there has been an enormous fragmentation in human experiences—politics, theology, sociology, technology, natural science, literature. So wholism, as a notion, is really a kind of profound human response to the unsatisfactory fragmentation of the oneness of human life."

Hilliard Jason, Jane's second husband and an internationally known physician and medical educator who created and directed the division of faculty of development at the Association of American Medical Colleges in Washington, DC, spoke at the symposium. Among other topics, he emphasized that we need professionals "who are alert to their own limitations and respectful of the strengths of others." "Yet," he added, "a great deal of what goes on in the medical education process focuses almost exclusively on the importance of having the 'right answers', rather than acknowledging the complexity of health care and the need for multiple perspectives on issues." He argued that we need doctors who are "aware of their own limitations and respectful of the views of patients, nurses, and others who are involved in the healthcare process." He called for demystifying medicine and education, and empowering patients, students, and clinical colleagues so that we can move closer to having an authentic team approach to patient care.

Two of Granger's daughters were at the national symposium. Jill was a member of the WHC staff. Jane accompanied her husband and colleague, Hill Jason. Being in medical education herself, Jane was also interested in the presentations. When Hill and Jane married in 1976, Jane and her sons moved to Washington DC, where Hill was based. Jane, who had been on the faculty of the department of family medicine at the University of Miami since 1972, joined the faculty of the medical school at George Washington University. Years earlier Jane had told Granger she did not want to become a physician. Later, however, she became interested in working in a setting that focused on educating physicians to relate sensitively and effectively to the whole person, so Jane did her doctoral studies in psychology and education and worked in the new field of family medicine.

Jane, Jill, and Hill were impressed with the way Granger shared the spotlight with his staff. As the founder and senior person of the WHC project, it would have been natural for him to be center stage throughout the conference. While he did make important contributions they felt that he clearly chose to give the younger members of his staff an opportunity to shine.

Lessons about Facilitating Change

In 1978, Granger wrote a document for the W. K. Kellogg Foundation titled, "Dissemination of Wholistic Health Centers." In it he reflected on the process in which he and his colleagues had been engaging and some of the lessons they were learning.

> We had an idea whose time had not quite come but was in the process of becoming ... so we had to give most of our attention to educating the community regarding wholistic health care and what we were trying to accomplish.
>
> Knowing that any new idea takes anywhere from 10 to 20 years to come into full bloom, we were fortunate to have foundation help during the formative years when the people were responding to the concept with mild enthusiasm but were not quite ready to invest their own money or lives in this kind of medical care. We were, in a sense, fortunate to be involved in this project at a time when there was growing dissatisfaction with the impersonal, technologically-oriented medical care by physicians. The fact that physicians were seeing patients for such brief times and charging such high rates also created a desire to find another pattern of health care.

In talking about his dreams for Wholistic Health Centers, Granger revealed some of his strategies as a change agent:

I am aware that it will take the approval of the American Medical Association (AMA), the large denominations of churches, and the American Hospital Association to give it the impetus to happen. This is one of the reasons why I feel it is important to do new things within the context of the establishment. We have purposely taken no steps forward without consulting people in the AMA, in medical education, and in churches (including bishops) concerning what we intended to do.

We have felt that it would be wrong to stand on the outside and shout epithets at our elders in the establishment ... We think our dreams are more certain of success when each step along the way is approved by people in positions of trust in the establishment.

Granger admitted that he and his colleagues had to look hard before they found a few key people in establishment positions who were willing to listen to what they had to say and then offer encouragement. When these people spoke quietly but clearly on behalf of WHC, it took some of the sting out of the organization's radical image and resulted in less resistance from other establishment leaders.

We regret that our image has been tarnished somewhat by newspaper writers lumping us together with other "holistic" people who espouse more radical concepts. While we believe in much of their basic philosophy, our method of practice is more traditional. We have found it necessary to stress our traditional side so that we attract a cross-section of people. We must meet them first where they feel comfortable and then introduce them to methods of treatment that deal with more than just the physical dimension.

Granger 's biggest disappointment was that most physicians, with the exception of a few in family practice and preventive medicine, were not enthusiastic about Wholistic Health Centers. Even those who were interested felt that the centers were still sufficiently "far out" that they would lose stature with their colleagues in medical practice if they were to join such a "radical movement."

Granger was more hopeful about the younger generation of physicians. Since the WHCs opened, a few medical students and residents had been working at WHCs as part of their elective clinical experiences. For the most part, the medical students and residents who spent time at the WHCs were disillusioned with their education and were seeking settings where they could learn and practice whole person medicine.

Dr. Paul Holinger reported that spending time at the Center, both as a medical student and then as a resident, enabled him to see a model that welded together the many aspects of whole person care. He said that that the Center was a unique setting in which people not only espoused, but were dedicated to, practicing principles that he considered vital to good health care delivery.

Despite these obstacles, the approach of the WHCs began to have impact beyond the local communities they served. G. Scott Morris was a young Methodist seminary student at Yale, intending to go to medical school after seminary. Then he would open a clinic to treat the whole person, body and spirit. Since his boyhood, he had been convinced the church did not do enough to live out the healing dimension of the gospel. While attending seminary at Yale, he was drawn to the chaplain of the medical school who also taught in the divinity school. One day Morris found in the chaplain's office a small publication—less than 20 pages—called *How to Start a Church-based Health Clinic* by Granger Westberg. Before this, Morris had not heard of Granger. Now he couldn't wait to meet him, thrilled with the discovery that others were doing what he hoped to do as well. The next day, he was on the phone with Granger.

During the summer after that academic year, Morris went to Illinois to meet Granger and see how the clinic worked. Later, as a medical student, Morris spent a month in the Hinsdale center absorbing all he could about Granger's approach to whole person health care. After medical school and residency in family practice, Morris's calling drew him to Memphis, Tennessee, to offer health care to the uninsured working in low-wage jobs, with equal commitment to wellness in body and spirit for all people. In 1987 he opened the Church Health Center, which harnesses the strengths of the faith community and does not rely on government funding. Over the course of its history, the Church Health Center has grown from one small clinic in a rehabbed house, with a couple of treadmills for its wellness program, to providing a medical home to 55,000 uninsured patients. Right from the start, the Church Health Center has funded wellness and health promotion as robustly as clinical care, and Morris continues to tell the story of his discovery of Granger's pioneering work to the young doctors now in his growing sphere of influence.

Impressed by Nurses

Granger also was increasingly impressed with nurses. He recalled, "At that time people in the nursing professions had been talking about wholistic approaches for at least two decades. Their textbooks and journals were filled with recommendations of how to humanize health care. I found nurses to be the most enthusiastic audiences I had occasion to speak to."

When Granger returned to Chicago, Helen Grace, then dean of the College of Nursing at the University of Illinois, gave him encouragement and advice. After the WHC was established in Hinsdale, she was one of the first people Granger invited to speak to the staff. Nurses were among the early volunteers at Wholistic Health Centers. When patients came to the WHCs, nurses typically introduced them to the WHC and served as coordinators of their care.

Student nurses did electives at the WHCs where their nursing supervisors worked with them on the skills needed for being effective patient advocates and health educators. Most nursing practicums tended to be in fast-paced, technically-oriented hospitals, so students were appreciative that the staff at the Centers encouraged and supported them in taking time with patients.[1]

Although Granger was enthusiastic about the contributions of nurses, his strategy at this time was to work through the traditional medical structure. Within that structure he sadly thought that the nursing profession was not yet in a position to help shape high-level policy decisions.[2]

Granger's Rangers

In 1979, five more Wholistic Health Centers were established. In the Wholistic Health Center network, there were now 13 physicians, 16 registered nurses, 13 pastoral counselors, 17 allied health professionals and administrators, and a host of trained volunteers. In his 1979 annual report to Kellogg, Granger was more optimistic than he had been the previous year:

> I see great potential for change and growth to take place within the present medical establishment and within present church and corporate establishments regarding a more wholistic approach to health. I admit it is slow, but I think it is sure. It is much like trying to change things within a democracy, but I also prefer to work within a democracy.
>
> For 35 years I have been needling my colleagues within the church and within medicine until they hate to see me coming. It hasn't been altogether pleasant; but now, after all these years, we are beginning to see a breakthrough occurring.

Minister and doctor and nurse are meeting ... in a way that is recognizing the need for a wholistic approach dealing with body, mind, and spirit.

In 1979 the Rev. Bill Peterson joined John Riedel in the national office for Wholistic Health Centers, both serving as "Granger's rangers." Bill recalled:

Granger would go out on the road speaking, getting people excited about Wholistic Health Centers. Sometimes we weren't even sure where he was. But shortly after he left a place, we'd get a call saying, "Granger Westberg was here a week ago. We've got a group together and we're ready to start a Wholistic Health Center." John and I would then go to the church and help the group decide what would work in their setting. Sometimes a Wholistic Health Center was feasible; sometimes they would have to come up with a form that would work better in their setting.

Granger would get people cranked up. He didn't choose to help people follow through with all the details and maybe he even felt he didn't have the ability to do that well. He knew what he could do, and when he was done, he left. But he always left people wanting more.

Before long an overwhelming number of people wanted to visit the WHC or to have WHC staff members visit them. In 1980, the national office of Wholistic Health Centers set up quarterly meetings to which the staff invited physicians, nurses, pastors, hospital administrators, and others who wanted to learn about the concepts and approaches of the WHCs. Granger and the other staff members made presentations, did role-plays, and conducted discussions.

Most of the attendees decided that creating a Wholistic Health Center was too big an undertaking for most churches. John Riedel remembered:[3]

It would have been nice to have many more centers but with the problems of insurance reimbursement, physician salaries and all, that was hard to achieve. Even so I think that we had an important impact on many of the people who came to the conferences or heard Granger and others speak or read the material written by the center staff.

Many health professionals incorporated what they learned into their practices. They did such things as include meaning-of-life issues into their care of patients or begin to work as a team. All of the centers were, in a sense, laboratories trying different approaches. They freely shared what they learned.

John was amazed at how Granger maintained his optimism despite some real challenges: "Granger could pick a dream and hang with it. He had a wonderful combination of idealism and altruism along with the ability to hang in there and get others excited and see his dream through. You don't come across that very often in life … Granger took joy of living to heart. There was always a bounce to his step. Sometimes when he and some of the Wholistic Health Center family were walking together, he'd start running and urge us to follow."

The national office supported the Wholistic Health Centers by such activities as creating publications and conducting an annual three-day retreat. Bill recalls:

We had a very strong network. For five years (1979–84), we gathered annually at George Williams College Camp at Lake Geneva. We'd tell stories, lick our wounds, celebrate what we had accomplished, and have fun. One of the reasons that I think physicians and others took time to come year after year was that they wanted to have time with Granger. Being with Granger helped them renew their energy and commitment.

Teams from each clinic would present something about their

work. It was almost always humorous. I remember Granger laughing so hard at how his dream actually turned out. Granger's laughter encouraged us to have a sense of humor and perspective. He reminded us that there was no precise formula and that to some extent we had to make things up as we went along.

Granger was always an advocate for the spiritual dimension. If we would get too medical or too psychological, he would remind us about issues of faith, values, and ethics. He kept bringing us back to those issues.

During one of the conferences on Lake Geneva, Granger invited Bill Peterson, John Riedel and others to take a ride in his motorboat. Bill recalls:

The boat had to be taken out of the water when it wasn't being used because if it was left in the lake it would fill up with water and sink. For Granger this was not a problem. He couldn't understand why other people saw it as a problem because he simply winched the boat up out of the water when he wasn't using it.

Having heard the stories about the boat, we were a little hesitant to join him, but he said, "Don't worry about it," so we went out with him. As we rode along, though, water did start seeping in, so we expressed our concern. He said, "This boat is kind of like life. As long as you keep moving, you're okay. If you stop, you're sunk."

Granger's leaky boat illustrated a lot about him. He seemed to see possibilities where other people saw problems. When one of his ideas and projects played out or was institutionalized, he was already on to other ideas, still traveling on, like his boat.

Health Cabinets for Churches?

While Jill was working at the national office of WHCs she attended a small, experimenting Lutheran church. The minister, Jack Lundin, was an ardent supporter of Granger's work. He wanted to have a WHC in his church, but his church, like so many churches, had neither the space nor the money needed for a WHC. Jack thought up an alternative: a health cabinet. His logic was that if homes have medicine cabinets then churches should have health cabinets. In a church community that thrived on new ideas, the health cabinet took off.

Jill was among the 18 people who showed up for the first meeting. Jill remembered, "First we acknowledged what we were already doing to promote health, such as sharing joys and concerns during worship and taking meals to the folks who are sick. Each of the 18 people also had new ideas they wanted to implement. Eventually I chaired this committee and shared my church's experiences with Dad and my co-workers at the Wholistic Health Center. Naturally Dad suggested that I test out the idea in other congregations."

Jill graduated from college. After a break of a couple of years, she wanted to continue her education and find some way to pursue her interest in the potential of health cabinets. Jill found a progressive graduate school that accepted her proposal for a combination of practical and theoretical study in faith and health.

Jill envisioned the health cabinet as a group of volunteers who are committed to the healing ministry of the church. This included helping individuals and families become more responsible for maintaining and improving their own health and the health of their community.

According to Jill, health cabinets could work in three main ways. First they could sponsor health-related activities through already existing structures, such as worship, Sunday school classes, and youth groups. Second, they could sponsor new health-related activities. Third, they could assess the "overall health and 'unhealth' in the life of the whole congregation," and then work at ways to support what is healthy and to "turn the 'unhealth' around."

Through Wholistic Health Centers, Inc., Jill was successful in securing a grant from the Wheat Ridge Foundation to test the health cabinet model and write a start-up manual. Jill:

> After a year all the pilots exceeded my expectations. They were a natural extension of what we at WHC were doing and a model for churches that wanted a health ministry but couldn't have a WHC. The president of the local United Church of Christ hospital system, then called Evangelical Health Association (EHA), loved the concept. He hired me to promote health ministry in the 80 UCC churches connected with their five hospitals. After the success I'd experienced, I expected that "selling" health cabinets to other churches would be a snap. Boy, was I wrong.

Quickly Jill learned that members of many congregations were overworked and not excited about setting up yet another committee. For three years at EHA, Jill tried many strategies for helping churches commit to trying the model.

Jill recalled, "I finally chose instead to be a full-time mom and part-time writer. I felt I had seen the last of health cabinets. What I failed to realize was that the Parish Nurse Project was to play an important role in fanning the flames on the health cabinets."

Chapter 19

Retirement or Refirement?

In 1981, the W. K. Kellogg Foundation staff members were planning to visit the national office of Wholistic Health Centers, Inc. regarding the renewal of a grant. Bill Peterson recalled:

> We were expected to do a presentation, so we suggested creating impressive slides and charts. Granger, however, said that we should just write down that information and give it to the people from Kellogg. Instead of doing a slide and chart presentation, he said that he just wanted to talk.
>
> When the people from Kellogg came, we and our board sat with them in the church library. As Granger started to tell his stories and get everyone involved, a rung from his chair broke. We looked at him and each other, but he continued to talk. Then another rung broke. Still Granger kept telling his stories. Slowly the chair collapsed beneath him, sinking him to the floor. Gracefully and slowly, without missing a beat, Granger pulled over another chair, sat down, and continued talking. I'm sure that's why we got the second grant. I think that the people from Kellogg realized that anyone who could maintain focus while his chair collapsed beneath him had what it took to complete their project.

By late in 1981, there were 12 Wholistic Health Centers.[1] With few exceptions, the Centers were financially viable, thanks to a combination of fee-for-service payments from patients, support by local churches, physicians willing to accept relatively low salaries, and contributions from individuals and private foundations. As Granger had wanted, the WHCs were situated in low-, middle-, and high-income communities, in urban, suburban, and rural locations.

After interviewing Granger about the WHCs, in his nationally syndicated column that appeared in the *Chicago Tribune* Bruce Buursma wrote:[2] "Westberg acknowledges that each of the centers is free to develop its 'own personality' and convictions about health care. But he says the wholistic centers differ from conventional clinics in their emphasis on preventive health care and 'pastoral' counseling. 'There is a difference between pastoral care and psychology. We're not ashamed to talk about God. We believe Christ is the Great Physician.'"

Buursma asked Granger how the Wholistic Health Centers related to the holistic medicine movement, with its emphasis on alternative practices and mystical Eastern religious philosophies. Granger replied, "I sense they aren't talking about the same thing we are. I salute them for their willingness to test new ways to get at the cause and cure of illness. But I have tried hard to keep our project within the fold of traditional American medicine and religion. I'm just trying to get the church back in the business of living out the gospel message of health and salvation."

Retirement?

Granger was now past the usual age of retirement. He cared deeply about the Wholistic Health Centers but wondered if it was time to change his relationship with the enterprise and free up his salary so those badly needed funds could be used to move the programs forward. Researchers evaluating the Wholistic Health Centers had concluded that the WHC model was "simultaneously orthodox and radical" and was working "within the context of organized medicine." The project was deemed successful but costly.

In some notes that he wrote to himself Granger said,[3] "I have chosen the most trustworthy young people anyone could ever find. They are all gifted in their respective areas of competence. They are not youngsters—one has almost grown children—and all have years of experience in back of them. I am not needed by them on all decisions. I could be gone for three months and everything would go along fine. The board of directors trusts the team and seems willing to go along with their dreams."

Granger also noted some issues that he wondered if others might be better able to deal with:

1. Inflation is the number one problem. Whereas we once could put a new center together for about $50,000 to $70,000, now we need $100,000, and this scares off congregations.

2. We have not been able to train doctors, as we had hoped, in the wholistic ways of practice. This is partly due to being part of the University of Illinois, which has not been able to get its family practice department off the ground.

3. Our idealistic model, which at its best with the right staff works so well, flies in the face of every means that doctors' offices use to make money; that is, we do not order lots of tests, we take time with patients, etc.

4. Many of the things we did early, such as educational classes, are now being done by an increasing number of groups, such as HMOs, some doctors' groups, hospitals, churches, counseling centers, etc.

In the fall 1981, after spending the previous winter working at the University of Arizona, Granger wrote in *Wholistic Wellspring*, the newsletter of the Wholistic Health Center network:

This is to tell you that, now that I've reached 68, I've decided to retire so that Helen and I will be free to take longer vacations and three-month sabbaticals in the winter in places like the University of Arizona College of Medicine.

The Board of Directors has voted me the title Founder/ President Emeritus. I will continue as a consultant and will spend my time developing new projects. This will free me of administrative responsibilities, which will be in the hands of our very competent young Executive Director, Richard King, with John Riedel and Bill Peterson continuing their fine work in development and education.

Following Granger's retirement, Richard M. King, the WHC's business manager, wrote:[4]

The true strength of any organization lies not in its plans nor in its edifices nor even in its purposes. Its true strength lies in its leadership ability ... Granger Westberg has dreams and ideas that will transcend their place in time and history. Few people are blessed with such a gift. It is naive to believe that his retirement will not have some impact on the wholistic movement. At the same time, however, the skills of his past leadership has given direction to the hundreds who will now take up the task.

Bill Peterson had another view of Granger's retirement: "Granger decided that he was going to retire. I'm not sure why he wanted to. Maybe he was tired of doctors' attitudes. So we decided to have a big party and do some fundraising. We created the Westberg Institute. Bob DeVries and the whole crowd came to the party. A special song was even written about Granger and his Chris Craft boat. Two weeks later, he showed up at his desk. That didn't surprise any of us. He said, 'I still have work to do. I don't know what people do in retirement.'

I think he retired two more times after that. Finally I think he just gave up on retirement."

Prior to Granger's first attempt at retirement, Louis J. Kettel, dean of the School of Medicine at the University of Arizona, heard Granger speak in 1980 at a medical meeting in Chicago. Granger: "After my talk, Lou, who knew that I was retiring, said, 'I'm interested in what you're doing. I wonder if you'd like to come down to Tucson and be a visiting professor during the winter quarter. You could be in the department of family medicine where you could share your stories with scores of young doctors.' Of course, I couldn't turn down that offer."

In January of 1981, Granger and Helen traveled to Tucson where Granger was based in the department of family and community health chaired by Dr. Anthony Ventura. Helen visited with her older sister, Elizabeth, and Elizabeth's family who lived in Tucson. Granger saw this as an opportunity to listen to young doctors and to talk with them about wholistic health. Granger spent time with students and faculty both at the family practice center located in the medical center and at another family practice facility located in the community. Granger particularly enjoyed the daily interdisciplinary case conferences involving 15-20 physicians and other professionals.

In the summer of 1981, Granger wrote the following about his experience in Arizona in the Wholistic Health Centers, Inc. newsletter, *Network News*:

> The discussions were far ranging, all persons contributing their particular insights. I didn't open my mouth the entire first week (unusual for me!). Then, little by little, I began to feel accepted by the participants who I joined in making hospital rounds and seeing patients in the outpatient clinic. I would comment on the spiritual dimensions of the wholistic approach to the problem under consideration. They were unusually receptive to such discussions, so receptive that I am now planning to redirect

my efforts on the home front here in the Chicago area. I hope
to spend most of my time away from administration and into
participating in similar family practice residence conferences
in Chicago-area hospitals.

... If our wholistic concepts are ever to be understood and
integrated with good medical practice, we must introduce
medical residents to them early in their training. And they
should have opportunities to engage in open debate concerning
these principles throughout their three years of residency. In
addition, they should be able to participate in seeing patients
in settings devoted to wholism.

Granger felt this could happen most easily if Wholistic Health
Centers were located near medical schools and residency training
programs. He declared, "With these goals in mind, I've got my work
cut out for me for the next 30 years."

Granger and Helen had such a wonderful sabbatical in Arizona
in 1981 that they returned for three consecutive winter sabbaticals
after his official—but not very effective—retirement.

Meanwhile, in early 1984 the national office of Wholistic Health
Centers, Inc. had to close. The national office was not proving to
be financially viable, particularly in the difficult economic times
nationally. The individual Wholistic Health Centers, however, were
still viable as separate corporations, so the staffs at the centers joined
together and formed the Wholistic Health Network.

In 1986 in his "Notes from the President" in the *Network News*,
Granger, at age 73, wrote: "Some of you know that I tried to retire
but it just didn't work. My heart is wholly in things wholistic. So I'm
back working two-thirds of my time and loafing for a third of the
time. My wife, Helen, and I are doing many of the things we didn't
have the time for before. I can strongly recommend the 2/3–1/3
plan as a great way to retire ... I am so grateful for what you all have
been doing to make our Wholistic Centers worthy of praise. Some

have recently expanded existing facilitates and others have moved to new offices to meet their growing needs."

The WHC model continued to inspire others to create new centers, using similar models. Granger was pleased with the progress, but he also felt that others probably were better equipped than he was to deal with such problems as the increasing cost of creating and maintaining WHCs. Granger continued to be an advocate and spokesperson for WHCs, but he was putting even more energy into a new dream that emerged from his work with the WHCs.

Chapter 20

Nurse in the Church

In early 1983 during the winter quarter, Granger was teaching at the University of Arizona. One morning he was drinking coffee with some faculty members in the department of family and community medicine. They were talking about how they might help a local congregation see that it could play an important role in helping people to stay well. Just then the dean of the medical school, Louis Kettel, walked by. Someone said, "Let's get the dean in here and talk."

Granger:

> After talking with us a while, Lou said, "You know, I've been thinking, we should start a clinic in my church. It's right across the street from the medical school. The problem, though, is that there probably isn't room enough for a clinic." I agreed because I had been at his church, Our Savior's Lutheran Church. Then Lou said, "You say so many wonderful things about nurses and how they've become the glue that hold the clinics together. How would it be if we put just one nurse on our staff and see how that worked?"
>
> Vicki Young, a physician assistant who was a former Roman Catholic nun, was sitting near us. "I've been overhearing your conversation she said, "I want to be the first candidate for that job.'"

Granger had actually being toying with this "nurse-in-the-church" idea for several years.

In a relatively short time, the Our Savior's congregation approved the project.

Lou, with help from Granger, got $40,000 in funding for the project from a Phoenix, Arizona-based foundation. Lou also talked with members of the county medical association to assure them that the clinic would not take patients away from them; that it would provide supplemental care and referrals, not primary care.

After the winter quarter was over, Helen and Granger returned home to Downers Grove, Illinois. It was taking a while for everything to fall in place so Vicki could begin her work, but Granger, the eternal optimist, was hopeful.

Even before Vicki had begun her work in Tucson, Granger was talking about also putting nurses in other churches around the country. In August of 1983, Bruce Buursma of the *Chicago Tribune* reported the following in his syndicated column:[1] "Granger Westberg is stepping up his long-standing crusade to wed religion and science, to transform church sanctuaries into clinics for both spiritual souls and physical bodies." Buursma quoted Granger as saying, "When Christ sent the disciples out, he told them to go preach and heal. The church has been doing a lot of preaching, but we haven't done nearly as much healing as we should."

Buursma reported that Westberg "a 70-year-old ordained Lutheran pastor" is "prescribing a simple remedy for that religious ailment: a nurse in every church as a 'minister of health' on the parish pastoral staff. His prescription is to be tested next month in a pilot project at Our Saviour's Lutheran Church in Tucson, Arizona." Buursma said that Granger had also set his sights on having similar "nurses in churches" programs in other cities, such as Chicago, Seattle, and Denver, contending that preventive health care is the most important service US churches can provide. He quoted Granger:

A large percentage of Americans are kept well by the relationship to their community of faith. If we could have nurses easily available in churches, we would pick up the early cries for help that we're now missing … A nurse is needed more as a kind of pastoral figure than strictly a medical technician. I see many nurses having this pastoral quality, but it is going to waste because they're kept busy doing the technical things.

Roles of the Parish Nurse

In his conversation with Buursma and earlier in communications with others,[2] Granger said that as a minister of health the church nurse would have a position on the parish staff similar to any associate minister. The nurses' work would vary depending on the needs of the congregation and community. Most nurses, however, would have the following four roles.

Health educator for the congregation and community. The nurse would lead, or bring in others to lead, courses, seminars, and workshops for the congregation on a wide variety of health-related topics, such as health maintenance, disease prevention, early detection through screening, the role of emotions in illness, and the interrelation of body and soul. She would "raise the understanding of how the spirit is related to health and wholeness."

Personal health counselor. Primarily with members of the congregation, but also with some nonmembers, the nurse would:

1. Provide a professional listening ear.
2. Do some assessment of health problems.
3. Recommend and/or provide minor health care measures, or refer people to a physician and/or community support services, as needed.
4. Serve as a role model of good health concepts.
5. Educate individuals in specific ways they could take better care of themselves.

Facilitator and teacher of volunteers. The nurse would be a catalyst, helping members of the congregation see how they can be more active in the health care ministry. For example, she could seek out people in the congregation who are empathic, good listeners, and willing to listen to others who were in pain, and she would provide these people with opportunities to enhance and use their skills. In addition, the parish nurse would call upon other health care professionals to teach courses in their areas of expertise and help her do screening and assessment.

Liaison person and organizer of support groups. The nurse would open doors for parishioners into the complex medical world. She also would identify support groups and other resources outside the church and refer parishioners when appropriate. If groups focused on needed topics, such as weight loss, divorce, and loss and grief, were not available in the community, she would organize and even facilitate them.

Kellogg: An Old Friend

Dr. Edward Lichter, Granger's chairperson at the University of Illinois School of Medicine, again supported Granger's ideas. In September 1983, he sent Helen Grace,[3] then on the staff of the W. K. Kellogg Foundation, a draft of a proposal for "church nurses." In his cover letter, Ed, referring to the content of the proposal, wrote: "It seems like a familiar refrain that you and Granger and I spoke about more than 10 years ago. I think the times have finally caught up with the idea, and we are ready to try it out. ... Granger is very excited about this project and wants to start it next week. I think it should take a little longer to get it set up. ... I think the project is 'doable' and important for extending primary prevention into the community."

In the proposal, Ed and Granger wrote that in their 10 years of work on the Wholistic Health Centers they encountered many congregations that were interested in having Wholistic Health Centers but could not set one up because the financial burden was too great or they did not have adequate physical space. Several churches, however, indicated that they could support a "church nurse."

Kellogg's response was enthusiastic. Over the years they supported the creation of a solid foundation for what was to become a parish nurse movement.

In November, when Granger and Helen returned to Tucson for their fourth winter sabbatical, Vicki Young was officially working for Our Saviour's Church as their minister of health. Although Vicki was a physician assistant, she was helping to pioneer the roles that later would be assumed by nurses. Vicki worked under the supervision of Ron Pust, MD, also a member of Our Saviour's. Vicki, who as a nun had taught for 20 years before becoming a physician assistant, led health care classes for congregational groups. She also had an open clinic 16 hours a week. A journalist quoted Vicki as saying,[4] "People who want to do self-care feel free to discuss it with me. Sometimes after patients have been to their physicians, they'll come to me with questions. Then I try to teach them how to communicate with their doctors."

The journalist also quoted Dean Lou Kettel who observed:

Vicki supports patients and takes time to help them sort out the issues of their health. She is filling a void in our very complicated medical system that is specialized and costly. What Our Saviour's Church is doing saves patients and the health system money and keeps people closer to wellness than sickness. While any social organization could perform such a service, the church is an environment with lots of support available. It is something the church has the right and obligation to do.

A difficult question is whether such a program can be sustained in a congregation. Is it really cost-effective in the church? Will people accept it as having the same value as I perceive it to have?

Chapter 21

Flight Test

Back home from Arizona and eager to put nurses in churches, Granger visited his friend, George Caldwell, who was president and chief executive officer of the Lutheran General Health Care System. Granger: "As I was waiting for the elevator to go up to the floor where I was going to meet with George, the elevator door opened. There was Anne Marie Djupe, one of the very bright, enthusiastic nurses who worked with us at the Wholistic Health Center in Hinsdale. We hugged and she asked, 'What are you doing here?' When I told her about my dream, she said, 'Oh my, I'm very interested.' And indeed she was.

"I told George about my dream of putting nurses in churches. He felt the project was congruent with the hospital's mission. He said, 'Granger, let's do it.'"

Later Caldwell reported that he was delighted and flattered that Granger approached him and Lutheran General. He had been an admirer of Granger since the late 1950s when, as a young hospital administrator, one of his first assignments had been to do the administrative work for a symposium for doctors and clergy in Rockford, Illinois, at which Granger was the keynote speaker. He remembered:[1] "Granger's notion of wholeness and health care and medicine and ministry struck a response in me. I kept track of Granger and his work."

Recalling his first conversation with Granger about the Parish Nurse Project, Caldwell said, "The notion of a nurse in the church was easy for me to comprehend, easy for me to support and to assign resources to. First, it fit the mission of Lutheran General. Second, I thought it made good business sense. Third, it fit my personal notion of what the church is about and ought to be."

Granger: "It took about a year and a half to get the Parish Nurse Project underway. Because the project combines several disciplines, we had to decide in which department of the hospital it belonged. In the end, it was decided that the parish nurses would become part of the division of pastoral care, headed by the Rev. Larry Holst. That department had a natural affinity with congregations and had been including lay people in their regularly scheduled clinical education courses. The Parish Nurse Project would also have a close association with the division of nursing of the hospital."

In reflecting on his work with Granger, Holst recalled,[2] "I have a great deal of respect and admiration for Granger. He was very easy to work with and open to new ideas. Even though this was his vision, he was very willing to have other people add to it and redefine and reshape it a bit. As long as he wasn't losing the kernel or heart of the vision, he was willing to adapt."

Granger conceptualized the Parish Nurse Project as "an action-research project that places nurses on the staffs of congregations as 'ministers of health' to work alongside pastors and others who are dedicated to a wholistic ministry."[3] The presence of the nurse, Granger thought, could "remind people that the church is interested in whole persons—mind, spirit, and body."[4]

Pilot Test of Parish Nursing

Finally, Granger got the go-ahead to do some pilot testing of an action project in which six congregations would each hire a part-time nurse. It was agreed that the churches could be of many different denominations. Granger:

In deciding which churches to invite to participate in the project, we had to consider that each church would have to find about $10,000 or $11,000 a year for the salary of a half-time nurse. For the first two or three years, this limited us to large churches in affluent neighborhoods.

I visited some 20 large churches and told the story of the parish nurse program. There was almost immediate interest from every church. First I met with the pastor, then with smaller groups, such as the social ministry committee, members of the church council and groups of health professionals. Right away many people, especially the nurses, understood the merits of the idea and got excited about it. With this kind of interest, I thought that this was going to be an easy idea to sell.

Then, however, I had to confront the finance committees of the churches. They had other priorities. Ten thousand dollars a year was more than they cared to risk on such a radical idea. Soon I learned that churches do not have an item in their budget for "risk taking," which is too bad because churches should be open to testing out new ways of ministering to people.
I went back to the hospital and told them the bad news.

Again Lutheran General came to the rescue. I told George Caldwell that I felt that if churches could see the project in action, they would feel that they could afford a nurse. After consulting with others, he said that the hospital could offer churches a three-year contract whereby the hospital, during the first year, would pay three-fourths of the nurse's salary, one-half the second year, and one-fourth the third year. The following years, the congregation would pick up the entire cost. I was floored that the hospital would do this because it was a big outlay of funds.

George said,[5] "Congregations are not used to providing resources on matters of health and don't even see health necessarily as the church's business. I happen to see it as the church's business."

With this new commitment from Lutheran General, Granger went back to the churches. He remembered, "The finance committees began to squirm a little bit. Now they said that they were concerned about the nurses' benefit package. So I went back to the George. He suggested that we put the nurses on the staff of the hospital. That way they could have the same benefits that other staff received. The deal couldn't have been sweeter for the churches. Now they couldn't turn us down."

Meanwhile Lutheran General established the team that would provide leadership and educational opportunities for the nurses. Larry Holst was project administrator; Granger, the project developer and consultant. Anne Marie Djupe, the nurse who had worked at a WHC, had a key role in helping the nurses review and assess their work and in shepherding them in the evolution of their roles.[6]

Granger often attended six to eight meetings at each potential church. Finally he struck a deal with six congregations. On April 1, 1985, with the generous support from Lutheran General, six churches (three Lutheran, two Roman Catholic, and one Methodist) joined Lutheran General in a collaborative effort that put a part-time nurse on the staff of each church. Granger:[7]

> Each congregation was asked to organize a health cabinet made up of eight to a dozen members, who were interested in health, wholeness, and the spiritual dimensions of life. At this stage the cabinet's main responsibility would be to find the right nurse for that particular church. The cabinet was also to serve as the support group for the new nurse. Although she would report directly to the pastor in her daily work, this group of people could work closely with her as she began a type of ministry which the congregation had never before experienced.

Granger and his colleagues carefully thought through the kinds of capabilities they wanted candidates to have. In addition to good up-to-date nursing skills, they wanted nurses to be "sensitive listeners" and "spiritually mature." Granger and his colleagues advertised for nurse candidates through the usual channels. Within two weeks they had almost 30 candidates. This convinced them that there might be thousands of nurses looking for opportunities to use their talents in special forms of Christian ministry.

Granger found that the candidates were stimulated by the potential of a whole person approach. Most of them indicated their original motivation for going into nursing was strongly influenced by a desire to incorporate the spiritual dimension into their work. They were interested in a type of nursing that would allow them to be creative. Granger: "The hospital's nursing department screened candidates for nursing competencies. The pastoral care department sought to determine the candidates' potential for bringing the medical and spiritual dimensions together. Congregations made the final decision about the candidate they wanted as their parish nurse."

Meanwhile, the faculty, consisting of Granger, nurse Anne Marie Djupe, physician Greg Kirshner, and chaplains Flo Smithe and Lee Joeston, had to think through the educational program for the parish nurses. Granger:[8] "We immediately agreed that we didn't want to superimpose a curriculum on this first group of nurses, all of whom had a rich background of experience. Since their role, as we were now defining it, had yet to be tested, we could not pretend to anticipate their needs. Their course of instruction would have to be an evolving process with the nurses influencing its creation. Consequently, our structure was kept flexible from the outset."

The six nurses and churches in the first pilot project were Lois Coldewey at Lutheran Church of Atonement in Barrington; Mary Kay Frazier at St. Raymond's in Mt. Prospect; Sally McCarthy at Our Lady of Ransom in Niles; Saralea Holstrom at Our Savior's Lutheran Church in Naperville; Joan Linden at Grace Lutheran Church in La

Grange; and Laura Reichert at First Methodist Church in Park Ridge. The nurses met each week with Anne Marie Djupe and Granger for four or more hours. The other faculty joined them from time to time.

Granger: "In the classroom, we usually began by asking each nurse to tell us what kinds of experiences she had during the previous week ... The discussion and the emotions shared ... left all of us exhausted by the end of the class. But we were also exhilarated by hearing how these nurses were touching the lives of people in ways that had never before happened in those congregations. Growing out of these provocative discussions, a flexible curriculum gradually emerged."

For all of the nurses in the Parish Nurse Project, the first three months of work in the congregations primarily was a time to introduce whole person health care concepts. The nurses did health surveys, made presentations to various groups in the church, and communicated through the church newsletters. Some led sessions on health issues or invited others to do so. After these sessions, they were available for follow-up questions and private sessions.

A couple of nurses got off to a slow start that Granger and other reflected may have been due to inadequate preparation of key members of the church. Granger:[9]

> We who had worked with the project for many months often assumed that one long meeting with leading church members is all that it would take for them to understand and be committed to the project. We had to remember that for many people the idea of health care and wellness in the church was a radical idea ... they had to have it explained to them over and over again before they could explain it to other church members.
>
> We also learned that lay church leaders need to be involved early on in making the major decisions concerning the employment of a nurse on their staff. If the decision is made only by the pastor, it usually will not work.

The dedication and hard work of the parish nurses and their supporters paid off. The first year of the project was a success. All six nurses and churches wanted to continue. Since Lutheran General would be paying less of the six nurses' salary the second year, the hospital offered to add two more nurses and churches.

Recalling Granger's persistence in pounding the pavement and getting churches to commit to the parish nurse concept as well as Granger's continuing role in the project, Larry Holst said,[10]

> Granger is a grand guy. Everyone knows that he's a visionary, but a lot of people might not know about his tenacity and deep conviction. He isn't willing to come with an idea and hand it off. He comes with an idea and makes himself available to carry it out.
>
> ... If anything bothers me about Granger, it's that he's so continually euphoric. I can't imagine anyone being that happy about everything. I would feel like I was a walking depressive when I was with Granger.
>
> Anytime that I'd raise a potential problem, it was solved in Granger's mind, probably in 90 seconds.

Parish Nursing Takes Flight

Elsewhere in the country, the news about parish nurses had gotten out, largely due to the many talks Granger was invited to give about the Parish Nurse Project. Several parish nurse models were emerging. Some nurses were volunteers; others were salaried. Part-time or full-time salaries came from hospitals or churches or both. Nurses were in the inner city, the suburbs, and rural areas. Some nurses worked with one church; others worked with more than one church. Some were linked to hospitals; others were not. Although most nurses were carrying out the tasks that Granger had described (e.g., health educator, facilitator, and trainer of volunteers), each nurse was functioning in unique ways, depending on the needs of the people she served, the talent and expertise of each nurse, and the resources of the local church.

With his continuing dreams of ecumenism, Granger met with rabbinical associations in the hopes that nurses could be placed in synagogues. Nursing was not a strong part of the Jewish tradition, and there were relatively few Jewish nurses, so Granger stirred up interest but not much action. Granger hoped that people from other faith traditions outside of Christianity would see merit in involving nurses some day.

Meanwhile, Granger was thrilled that a significant proportion of the nurses and churches in the emerging parish nurse movement were Roman Catholic. Like Protestant nurses, Roman Catholic nurses are part of a nursing tradition that can trace its origins to the nursing done in homes by deaconesses of the early church and to the work of deaconess Fabiola who founded the first charity hospital in Rome about 300 AD. From that time forward, sisters have served as healers in many settings.

Chapter 22

Johnny Appleseed
of Parish Nursing

Even though the Parish Nurse Project was nicely underway, Granger enthusiastically continued seeking new converts. Ann Solari-Twadell was a nurse at Lutheran General Hospital working with the hospital's congregational health partnership program. She recalled: "We called Granger 'Johnny Appleseed' because he was charismatic and enjoyed speaking to groups. Granger would go into a town and talk about parish nursing. The people would get charged. They would want to know how to get the program going. But by then he was on to another show. So they tried to contact the nurses in the churches linked to Lutheran General to find out what they were doing." People interested in learning more about parish nursing overwhelmed the parish nurses in the six congregations. The six nurses could not develop the parish nurse role in their church and also respond to all the inquiries they were receiving about this new ministry.

Ann saw the need for a Parish Nurse Resource Center that could respond to national requests for assistance in developing this new professional model of health ministry. Ann approached her supervisor, the Rev. James Wiley, who was vice president of church relations, regarding the idea of starting a Parish Nurse Resource Center. Jim supported the idea, and Ann was able to take on the new work.

This center, with Ann as part-time director, had several functions:

1. Organizing and conducting educational programs, such as annual meetings, where prospective parish nurses and others could learn about the program, and where experienced parish nurses could share what they were learning.
2. Serving as a reference center for people who wanted information, including published materials, about the philosophy and work of parish nurses.
3. Consulting with churches, hospitals, agencies, and religious denominations who were interested in starting a parish nurse program.

The parish nurse program, now with eight nurses working in eight churches, was a separate entity. It continued to provide outreach for and was supported by Lutheran General. It also served as something of a laboratory for the national efforts in parish nursing.

The Resource Center quickly began developing a life of its own. Soon phone calls were coming to 312-696-8773, which spelled "my nurse." By January 1987, Ann, was spending 80 percent of her time as director of the Resource Center. As parish nursing grew to include sites in and resources from and for other countries, the name of the center was changed first to National Parish Nurse Resource Center and then to International Parish Nurse Resource Center (IPNRC).

A Handbook for Parish Nursing

Nurses, lay people, pastors, hospital administrators and others had been asking for written materials about parish nursing, so Granger with help from Jill, wrote a handbook titled, *The Parish Nurse: How to Start a Parish Nurse Program in Your Church*. The book pulled together a lot of what Granger had been talking and writing about for the past six years or so.[1] It included a chapter on the health cabinet, a concept that was being used in a growing number of churches.

At the heart of the handbook were eight steps for readers to consider if they wanted to develop a parish nurse program at their church:

1. Learn all you can about the program.
2. Communicate with the church pastor. "If the pastor is not interested in the idea, then there is little hope of success."
3. Educate the congregation. "To bolster your confidence, start with a group that will almost assure your success—nurses. Invite all the nurses from your congregation (and perhaps others) to an evening of discussion of the project. The response has uniformly been one of gratitude that somebody is finally recognizing the potential of nurses in preventive medicine and health education."
4. Form a health cabinet or committee. The cabinet can support the nurse's work and her continuing education.
5. Link up with a local hospital (an option). A partnership with a hospital can provide the parish nurse with regular support from other nurses and from chaplains.
6. Select a parish nurse. Let the pastor and members of the health cabinet take the major responsibility for this task.
7. Provide continuing education for the parish nurse.
8. Ensure that the parish nurse gets off to a good start by giving her adequate space and resources.

From the beginning of the project, Granger and his colleagues had been aware of the need for nurses to prepare themselves for the role of parish nurse and to continue learning throughout their careers. Parish nurses were expected to have an active nursing license in the state in which they were practicing. They were to keep their nursing skills and knowledge up-to-date, but they also needed to continue developing the knowledge and skills they needed as parish nurses. Granger:

When there are three or more nurses in a certain area, we think it is ideal for them to meet together on a regular basis both to support each other in their unusual responsibilities and to have medical experts sit with them to discuss medical and nursing aspects of their work. Parish nurses must deal with problems that nurses in other specialties may not encounter. These include, especially, the spiritual dimensions of illness. Because of this it would be well to include a chaplain or knowledgeable parish minister with the group on a continuing basis.

Granger and his colleagues suggested that nurses consider participating in the growing number of seminars in pastoral care and counseling sponsored by hospital chaplaincy departments. Although the courses were designed for local clergy, it was anticipated that ministers would be pleased when nurses attended because nurses would be able to contribute to the discussion of patient cases, including the physical and psychological issues. With their own real world stories (cases) and challenges, nurses might also want to participate in clinical pastoral education.

Granger Westberg Parish Nurse Symposium

A growing number of nurses did indeed want to prepare themselves to be parish nurses. In addition, nurses who were already serving as parish nurses wanted to network and share what they were learning. In response to these needs, and the request for information regarding this new health ministry, the Parish Nurse Resource Center held its first Granger Westberg Parish Nurse Symposium in September 1987. Martin Marty, the well-known Lutheran theologian and historian, was the keynote speaker. Seventy-eight enthusiastic parish nurses attended the session.

The growing number of parish nurses was reflected in the attendance of 135 people from 14 states at the second annual symposium in the fall of 1988. Following the symposium Granger wrote these "Reflections" in volume 4 of the *Parish Nurse News*.

The Symposium did my heart good. The fact that we had to move out of the small auditorium and use the big one said quite a bit about the progress we're making in telling the story of what parish nurses are doing in various parts of our country. At present we really don't know how many parish nurses there are. We do know that many nurses are volunteering their services to their local congregations, even if only for two or four hours a week ... I also know a lot of lay people, both men and women who are not nurses, who would like to help this program in many different ways ... I look forward to the next few years as 10,000 churches see the importance of placing parish nurses on their staffs.

Granger was very excited in 1989 when he heard that Lutheran General Health Care System was considering hiring Judith Ryan as senior vice president responsible for congregationally based health services and services for the aging. At that time Judith, a doctoral level nurse, was executive director of the American Nurses Association. Since 1988 she had served on the advisory board for the National Parish Nurse Resource Center. Judy reflected on her reason for serving on the council:[a] "I was attracted to the concept because of my own background in community health and because I believed that the focus of the Parish Nurse on the spiritual component of practice responded to nursing's historic professional stance. That is, nursing is the only health care discipline that has historically described the spiritual component to be part of its practice."

Thinking back on her first meeting with Granger, Judy said: "Immediately upon hearing of my potential appointment, Granger took me to breakfast at O'Hare Airport and 'grilled' me about my capacity to administer such a program! I literally knew him before I had met any of my other administrative colleagues at Lutheran!"

Granger was thrilled to find that Judy was "bright, articulate and very centered in the church." To Granger's delight, Judy accepted the position. From the beginning of her tenure, the parish nurse program (the nurses and parishes directly linked to Lutheran General) reported to her. Among other contributions, Judy always made sure there was a budget to support the parish nurse program, and she was a champion of the ongoing development of the professional role of the parish nurse. Shortly after Judy's arrival, Anne Marie Djupe became director of Parish Nursing Services.

Health Ministries Association

As interest in the parish nurse movement grew, Granger and many others felt that it would be useful to have a membership organization that included not only nurses but also ministers and others involved in healing ministries. The advisory board for the Parish Nurse Resource Center developed a proposal that resulted in the creation in 1989 of the Health Ministries Association (HMA), a national, nonprofit, ecumenical, interdisciplinary organization that Granger saw as an expansion of advocates for healing in congregations. An article in the *Parish Nurse News* stated that membership is open to "all people and institutions who are interested in the vision of the local congregation as the natural location for ministry to the body, mind, and spirit." It enables nurses "to join with other health care professionals, clergy, congregational members, educational institutions and health care institutions."

In 1990 Health Ministries Association received a three-year grant from the Kellogg Foundation to establish staff and begin national and regional programming to further the concept of parish nursing/ health ministries. HMA also received a "seed" grant from the Wheat Ridge Foundation (which was soon to be renamed "Wheat Ridge Ministries"). Nurse Mary Ellen Dyche and Rev. David Carlson were appointed co-directors of the organization.

Chapter 23

Traveling on a Single Track

Although he was getting on in years, Granger was continuing to travel and following his lifelong pattern of coming home earlier than planned. Later he wrote: "Helen and I have been very close friends for our 53 years. I love the wonderful home life she has made for our family. It's a standing joke at our house that I get homesick whenever I have to be out of town. They claim that I always figure out a way to take an earlier plane than my ticket shows."

Much of Granger's travels were on behalf of the Parish Nurse Project. On the road he gave talks to congregations, hospital staff, and other groups. Writing for one of the parish nurse newsletters, Granger said:

> I really don't like to travel. There is too much stress related to late planes due to "mechanical difficulties," weather delays, and parking problems at O'Hare Airport. Yet, once I get off the plane and meet the people who have invited me to talk about the Parish Nurse Program, I forget all about the discomforts of travel. I meet all kinds of wonderful people who care about the future of health care and see the churches of America as being able to contribute new insights, especially in the area of preventive medicine.

Initial Findings

People continued to want information about the Parish Nurse Project. Much had been learned since Granger and Jill wrote the handbook, so Granger, with help again from Jill, rewrote it with updated information, including reflections on the program's history and related issues. The book was called *The Parish Nurse: Providing a Minister of Health in Your Congregation.*[1]

In the introduction, Granger and Jill stated that after several years of experience and some systematic reflection and study of the "experimental" Parish Nurse Project, they could report four major findings.

1. Despite a national nursing shortage, congregations reported no difficulty finding unusual, qualified people with exceptional spiritual maturity. Many of these nurses had been disappointed by previous positions in hospital or clinics where there was no time for the kind of personal caring they felt patients needed so desperately.
2. The interest in parish nurses cut across societal groups, and programs were operating in urban, suburban, and rural areas.
3. Catholic and Protestant churches were working extremely well together.
4. Both religious and secular community hospitals were finding that parish nurses could be a link between them and their community. Hospitals who wanted to broaden their mission to include prevention and the first act of illness were realizing that parish nurses could help them in this endeavor.

Granger and Jill also reported that one of the studies of the parish nurse programs found that the organization and focus of the programs varied, depending on the gifts of the nurses and the motivation, needs, and resources of the congregations.[2]

The Kellogg Foundation continued to provide vital support in building a solid and carefully researched movement. In 1990 Kellogg provided more than three years of funding for documenting the parish nurse experiences and services, describing management tools, and establishing evaluation data. In 1994 Kellogg provided another substantial multi-year grant for studying and publishing findings about ways in which parish nursing services might be effectively linked into emerging community networks of care.

According to Judith Ryan, the results of the first Kellogg grant were used to publish the first workbook describing how to implement a parish nursing program: *Reaching Out: Parish Nursing Services*. This and other early publications were later used to guide the work of defining the practice, developing the curriculum for preparation in parish nursing, and setting the standards for credentialing the specialty practice of faith community nursing.

In 1995, the 650 nurses who attended the ninth annual Westberg Symposium included nurses from Canada, Germany, Sweden, Austria, and New Zealand. The parish nurse movement was a successful grassroots movement. Granger had been having difficulty making significant progress in the entrenched institutions of the church and health care, but these nurses were not waiting for their institutions. They were, in a very real sense, pioneers like Granger.

Granger opened his remarks to the symposium with a statement that his family could readily agree was true. "As most of you know, I have a single track mind. Everything I see or hear reminds me of parish nurses." Granger:

> You are blessing communities with your caring concern for all kinds of people. The people you serve are increasingly not only church members but also people who never thought the church had anything to offer them.
>
> ... I'm thrilled by the inspiring comments I constantly hear from parish pastors and their congregational members about what you nurses are accomplishing ... It has truly exceeded my fondest dreams of what can happen in any congregation,

large or small, rich or poor, when the professions of religion and health are yoked together. May God continue to bless your ministry.

Before becoming director of Parish Nursing Services, Anne Marie Djupe learned that she had breast cancer. Following treatment, she seemed to be doing well, but in 1993, the cancer reoccurred. Anne Marie's death, in 1995, was a loss for both Granger and Helen because Anne Marie was a friend as well as a colleague. Granger: "We are in debt to Anne Marie for setting a high standard for parish nursing. In many ways, she was the first parish nurse, because in the early days of the Wholistic Health Centers, she was already serving as a parish nurse. Anne Marie provided splendid leadership to parish nursing. She is deeply mourned by all of us."

In honor of Anne Marie, the Djupe family established an endowed lecture at the annual Westberg Symposium.

What Is a Parish Nurse?

As the number of nurses who wanted to become parish nurses continued to grow, there was increased demand for preparatory courses. In addition to the educational programs developed and offered by the National Parish Nurse Resource Center (NPNRC), other organizations also offered a variety of preparatory courses. Recognizing the need for guidelines, in 1994 the NPNRC brought together leaders in parish nursing from around the country and developed guidelines that were then published.[3, 4]

In 1996, under the umbrella of the National Parish Nurse Resource Center, Ann Solari-Twadell, directed a project in connection with Rosemarie Matheus of Marquette University and Mary Ann McDermott of Loyola University in which 35 experts, nominated from among thousands of parish nurses, systematically developed a basic standardized core curriculum for parish nurses and for the educators teaching this curriculum. To ensure nurses continue to keep pace with new research and best practices, the curriculum, which is now called *Foundations of Faith Community Nursing*, has been updated every five years since its original publication.

In 1997 the American Nurses Association recognized parish nursing as a specialty of the nursing profession. *Faith Community Nursing: Scope and Standards of Practice* was published the next year by the American Nursing Association and Health Ministries.[5] This book is also updated as the specialty grows.

In 1999 Ann Solari-Twadell and Mary Ann McDermott edited *Parish Nursing: Promoting Whole Person Health within Faith Communities*, a book about parish nursing[6,7] with a chapter by Granger titled, "A Personal Historical Perspective of Whole Person Health and the Congregation." The book also included such topics as parish nursing in rural and suburban communities, the community as client, parish nurse-physician partnership, parish nursing in diverse traditions, and educational preparation.

Granger was glad important work, such as curriculum development and reporting about projects was being done, and that such competent people were doing it. He knew this was not his area of expertise. Instead, to the extent that he was physically able, Granger continued telling the story of parish nurses and serving as their greatest supporter and advocate.

Chapter 24

An Elegant Affair ...
With the Lights Dimming

This account of Granger's remarkable life began with my (Jane) experience of walking my aging father into a crowded ballroom and discovering hundreds of people rising to their feet to welcome and thank him with their ovation. I have tried to write about Granger from a biographer's third person point of view. Allow me now, as we turn to the end of his life, to slip from my role as biographer to my experience as daughter once again.

In the late 1980s, Dad started having a tremor in one hand. Before too long, it became clear that Dad, like his brother and one of his uncles, had Parkinson's disease. Later he was also diagnosed with osteoporosis and chronic lymphocytic leukemia. With his lifelong optimism, he continued focusing on his dreams but the fatigue and the growing difficulty with speaking and moving made it impossible for him to keep up the pace that he had maintained most of his life. As the Parkinson's progressed, he said that one of his most difficult losses was his ability to smile.

Determined to keep on pursuing his missions and passions, Dad took walks every day and did exercises recommended for people with Parkinson's. One time when I was with him at a rehab center, he was supposed to practice walking backward. With a twinkle in his eyes, he turned to me and said, "Shall we dance?" Then to my delight and the delight of the physical therapists and others nearby, Dad and I danced.

To keep both his body and spirit alive, he took singing and piano lessons. Singing helped him project his voice, which increasingly was being reduced to a whisper. He finally got to have the piano lessons he had missed as a boy. The intentional movements of playing the piano countered the unintentional hand and arm movements of Parkinson's. As he had done all his life, Granger typically had classical music playing as he worked or rested.

Dad was not always an obedient patient. He was very reluctant to go to the hospital the few times that he had to do so. Once there, on at least one occasion, he checked himself out of the hospital against medical advice. Toward the very end, he also dismissed one or two home health providers, feeling that he and Mom could handle his needs. Unfortunately, that meant that Mom, now in her 80s also, had an overly heavy burden.

It was during this time, the last couple of years of his life, that Dad and I worked on his memoir, going through his papers, including early drafts of articles, letters, and speeches. He enjoyed rediscovering newspaper articles, photos, and other items that unlocked memories of events he had forgotten. As when he sang, when I recorded him telling his stories, he was able to reach deep inside of himself and find his voice.

I was living in Boulder, Colorado, because both my husband and I were professors at the University of Colorado School of Medicine. To stay in touch and to work on his memoir, Dad and I spoke by phone several times a week. Usually Dad was cheerful and spoke as loudly as he could. One day his voice was weak, and he seemed to be having trouble breathing. I asked, "Dad, would you like me to come to your house?" He whispered, "Yes." I checked with Mom, who was very worried about him. I took the next flight to Chicago.

When I got to Dad and Mom's home, John and Jill were there. Dad remained in the living room chair to greet me, but he was so sick that he let John help him to the bedroom. I said, "Dad, I think you have pneumonia. Would you like me to call an ambulance?" He nodded his head affirmatively. Earlier in life, Dad had recognized that pneumonia is "an old man's friend." He and I knew that left untreated, pneumonia can allow a patient to slip away relatively peacefully at the end of a long life.

With tears filling my eyes, I repeated, "Dad, I think you have pneumonia. Would you like me to call an ambulance?" He looked at me and nodded again.

When the ambulance crew arrived, they put Dad in the back of the ambulance. John, Mom, and Jill drove in the family car. I got to sit in the front of the ambulance. The ambulance had a special system that enabled the driver to switch red traffic lights to green so the ambulance could pass through. When Dad heard me exclaiming about this, he whispered to the medic who was attending him that he wanted to sit up front. The little boy in Dad was still alive and well even though his body was giving out.

In the emergency department, the doctor confirmed that Dad had pneumonia. Dad agreed to be treated. He was not ready to die. He had more that he wanted to do.

In November 1998, three months before Dad died, Parkinson's, leukemia, and osteoporosis had taken a toll on him. He was thin, bent over, and considerably shorter. Eating was difficult, and he could speak only haltingly. Nevertheless he was determined to attend an event at which Lutheran Social Service of Illinois was honoring him. My sister Jill and my brother, John, accompanied him. "It was an elegant affair with tables circling the dance floor," Jill remembers. Dad had been worrying about how he would accept the award. Since both walking and talking were difficult, he had been offered the option of acknowledging the award from his seat at the table. But when the time came for the award, it was clear Dad had decided to walk to the podium.

"John and I walked with him to the podium," Jill says, "helping him navigate over the maze of speaker wires. Then John and I sat back down at our table, leaving Dad on his own. They expected a short word of thanks after the award was handed to Dad, considering a few words at a time was all he could manage."

"What followed amazed me," Jill says. "He started into one of his familiar spiels about faith and health. I whispered to my husband, 'This is his 40-minute spiel.' He cut the speech short—perhaps it was 10 minutes. Then with another note of thanks he began walking a bit unsteadily back to the table. John and I both eyed the precarious wires on the floor and jumped up to steady him. A standing ovation followed."

Dad's health was deteriorating. After a short hospital stay, he agreed to go to a nursing care unit of a retirement home for a limited time. In the nursing unit he didn't get the intensive physical therapy he wanted. A week later, he was able to get into a rehab center. Jill agreed to accompany him.

While waiting for the medical car needed for transferring him to the rehab center, it dawned on Dad that this nursing care unit needed a parish nurse. He knew that once the administrator learned about the parish nurse concept, he would jump at the chance to hire a nurse, not just for the nursing care unit, but also the independent and assisted living sections.

Jill told me, "Dad insisted I push him in his wheelchair to see the administrator. How could I squelch his dream? Easy. I lied to him with only a bit of guilt. 'Dad, the offices are in the other building. If we go now, we'll miss the car.' I swear, that man never gave up."

At the rehab center Dad continued to make plans. He had it figured that our brother, John, who was happily ensconced in his own business, could work for this marvelous center.

One morning after about a week at the rehab center, Dad's vital signs crashed. He was rushed by ambulance to a nearby emergency room. Dad was lucid and understood the severity of his condition. He said to the ER physician, "Young man, you know your job well, so do what you need to do. But don't do a lot of tinkering because I'm about to meet my Maker."

Mom and John arrived soon after Dad was brought to the emergency room. After Dad's condition had stabilized, they decided to transfer him by ambulance to Good Samaritan Hospital in Downers Grove, where his family physician had privileges. That took almost eight hours for John to arrange. Meanwhile, while Dad was still on a gurney, Mom noticed Dad was trying to get up. When Mom asked him what he was doing, he said he wanted to do the exercises for his Parkinson's—something he had been doing every day.

When Dad was finally transferred and John was in the hospital room with him, a nurse told Dad that she had sent for his records. John remembers Dad smiling as best as he could and asking, "Are we going to play them?"

The hospital staff thought Dad's condition was stable. John went home and called Joan, Jill, and me to give us the news and to say that we didn't need to rush to the hospital. Hours later, though, John got a call from the hospital that Dad was unresponsive. He was dying. John called us again. I was in Miami, and it was too late for me to get a flight to Chicago that evening. Joan, who was in Oregon, was able to book a flight. Jill's husband was out of town so she stayed home with her children. John drove Mom to the hospital where they both stayed by Dad's bedside. Early in the morning the family minister arrived. John went home later in the morning; Mom stayed with Dad.

Joan arrived a little later in the morning. Jill came after taking her children to school. By that time Dad's breathing was labored. He was still unresponsive but as Joan said the Lord's Prayer, his lips moved, as if in prayer. John and I arrived a little later, but too late. He had died shortly before we arrived.

Chapter 25

Epilogue: Granger's Legacy

A **few days after Granger died in** February 1999, renowned Lutheran scholar Martin E. Marty wrote a letter to the Westberg family. About Granger, he said:

> He was the pioneer and mentor of us all in disciplines and practices that so many of us today take for granted and call our own. I've known him and his work since 1954 when I came to the University of Chicago. He never tired, never flagged, never lost cheer or hope or the ambition to make a difference in the arts of healing—both body and soul.
>
> Not many people can spend their late years seeing their inventions—I think of the parish nurse concept as an example— prospering and spawning offspring. Granger could.

Several years earlier, in January 1991, Shirley Barnes of the *Chicago Tribune* interviewed Granger, then 77, and described him as a "courtly gentlemen." She wrote, "For decades, Westberg spent much of his time stumping the country, speaking at major medical centers and conferences, trying to persuade theological leaders, medical students, and doctors of the wisdom of whole person care. He talked about how lifestyle, stress, self-esteem and grief offer vital clues to why people are sick and how pastors can help doctors spot these clues. Today, the message may sound old, but not when Westberg first broached the topic."

Ann Solari-Twadell, a vital person in the parish nursing movement now known as faith community nursing, captured the overarching theme of Granger's life and work. In a 1998 interview,[1] when Granger was still living, she said:

> His work has been foundational not only to parish nursing but to the broader piece of health ministry. He brought theological understanding. He brought that vision that it doesn't have to be the way it is today. He brought the understanding of the health care institution. He had that experience, and he certainly had the experience of the church. And he had tremendous energy, and drive, persistence, and fortitude
>
> Some people would look at Granger's life and say that he was into promoting whole person health. Yes, he was. But he was into way beyond that. More than anyone I've ever known, Granger was into the transformation of health care. I think that's the piece that people often don't understand. And if you don't understand that piece, then you miss some of the inspiration. He is about changing the way people think about health, the way they relate to health, and the role that the church can play in relating to health and the individual. He is into transforming the church as an agency of health. He is trying to provide an environment in which the individual can be transformed. He is also trying to transform our health care institutions.

During his multifaceted career, Granger sometimes encountered resistance to his ideas, but for those ideas in which he believed strongly, he just continued moving forward. In his later years, Granger had the joy of seeing how several of his major projects had endured and evolved, and were continuing to bear fruit.

Professional Chaplaincy

Granger's move into full-time chaplaincy was the first of several surprise twists in his career. Aware of the church's long history of healing ministries, he wanted to bring clergy back to the table as members of health teams. He spoke of concepts that were not common in his day, such as "health team" and "wholism." There were only a few Protestant chaplains in the early 1940s, and most of them were elderly and part-time. Granger, and colleagues such as Russell Dicks, thought it was important to increase the number of well-prepared, full-time chaplains. They created and called for more clinical pastoral education programs that enabled chaplains to develop capabilities needed to contribute to health teams and to the healing of patients and their families.

In 1946, under the auspices of the American Protestant Hospitals Association, Russell Dicks, then chaplain at Wesley Memorial Hospital in Chicago and Granger's good friend, invited hospital chaplains to meet about setting standards and strengthening their ministries within the institutions they served. The Association of Protestant Hospital Chaplains was born, later becoming the College of Chaplains and then the Association of Professional Chaplains. In the first year, Russell Dicks was president and Granger chaplain. For the second year, Granger was elected president.

Over the years, the College of Chaplains gave Granger several awards, including the Distinguished Service Award in 1992, and a new award called Christus in Mundo (Christ in the World) inaugurated to recognize contributions of "three giants of the pastoral care movement." All three recipients had served as president of the College. Following this recognition, Rev. Tom Droege, associate director of the Interfaith Health Program at the Carter Center, wrote to Granger:

> The reason for my writing other than saying I wish you could have been there to receive the recognition you so richly deserve from the College of Chaplains, is to share with you what I heard

over and over again, both in and out of the sessions. It always began something like this, "I got interested in this when I first met Granger Westberg." It got to be kind of a ritual refrain.

After I heard it a half dozen times, it hit me. If I trace my own biography back to the beginning of my long investment in the church and healing, I would have to begin the same way, "I got interested in this when I first met Granger Westberg. That was back in Billings Hospital [at the University of Chicago] as part of a class on ministry in the hospital, a class that medical students took alongside the Divinity School students. The medicine-religion conferences were classics that I still remember vividly."

Droege described how these events led to his career in religion and health and concluded, "So all of this is a way for me to say thank you for what you've done for me and thousands of others.

In 1996, at the fiftieth anniversary of the College of Chaplains, Granger was again honored for his pioneering work. Two years later the College merged with the Association of Mental Health Chaplains to form the Association of Professional Chaplains.[2] No longer linked only to Protestant hospitals, this enduring organization of more than 4,000 members is committed to interfaith ministry and to the professional practice of chaplaincy in a wide variety of settings. Its members, in Granger's legacy, improve health and well-being of the people they serve.

Good Grief

In Granger's most widely read book, *Good Grief*, he describes grief as a natural process that typically involves some well-documented stages. Granger saw grief not only in people experiencing the death of a loved one, but also in people dealing with different kinds of losses, including the loss of a job and the loss of a child in marriage (even in a good marriage). Originally published in 1962, by 1978 the book was selling so well that its publisher, Fortress Press, gave Granger its "Best-selling Author" Award. By 1985, the title had sold more than one million copies, and in 1987 the Religious Publishers Group honored Granger for this achievement. Rights to the book have been granted to publishers in numerous countries, including Australia, Brazil, Great Britain, Italy, Norway, Japan, South Korea, Sweden, Taiwan, and 20 Spanish-speaking countries in Latin America. In 2012, the publisher issued a fiftieth anniversary edition.

As of this writing, more than three and a half million copies of *Good Grief* have sold, casting a far-reaching legacy in the lives of people, many of whom likely never knew the scope of Granger's passion for supporting their well-being.

Academy of Parish Clergy

As early as 1963, Granger was convinced of the need for an American Academy of Parish Clergy on par with similar organizations serving other professions. *The Christian Century* published his proposal in 1965, and in 1968 he received funding that allowed him to take initial organizing steps. The organization took firm root. In 1975, the academy recognized Granger's visionary contribution with an award, and in 1991, he was honored as the "founding father of the Academy of Parish Clergy" with an honorary life membership in the academy.

The academy maintains a code of ethics and standards of competence in relationship building, communication, management, personal and professional growth, and celebration and worship. It also provides an annual conference with opportunities for continuing education, reflecting Granger's conviction that clergy must become more professional in order to engage as respected partners across disciplines that touch on the wellness of the whole person.

Real World Theological Education

First as a seminarian and later as a faculty member, Granger called for students to spend more time in real-world settings and far less time passively sitting in lectures. He also advocated for clinical education that focused on helping seminarians develop the skills needed for providing effective pastoral care. Over the years, thanks to the efforts of many people, Granger was able to see these changes occur, albeit slowly.

With his roots in the Lutheran church, Granger consistently approached his alma mater, Augustana Theological Seminary first, explaining his new ideas for theological education. On some occasions he got pushback, but he pressed on. One of Granger's dreams was for the various Lutheran seminaries to join and form a united seminary on a university campus where faculty and students could mix with faculty and students from other faiths and other academic fields. He especially wanted Lutherans on the University of Chicago campus and played a small role in sharing this vision with others. In the mid 1960s when the Lutheran School of Theology was built adjacent to the University of Chicago campus, Granger was thrilled. In later years the Lutheran School of Chicago honored Granger on several occasions.

Spirituality in Medical School Curricula

In the late 1950s, Granger was a pioneer in teaching classes in religion at a major secular medical school—the University of Chicago. He also taught some classes at Baylor Medical School. After leaving the Institute of Religion in Houston, Granger did not continue doing this work directly himself. He did have the joy of seeing others pick up this work. A survey in 2010 revealed that 90 percent of US medical schools had courses or content on spirituality and health in their curricula. However, despite acknowledging the importance of spirituality to patients, the majority of deans were uncertain about including spirituality in the curriculum and thought more content was not needed.[3] Clearly, Granger would think there is more work to do.

Wholistic Health Centers

In 1982, at age 69, Granger was honored by national leaders in theology, medicine, and philanthropy at a retirement banquet held at the Lutheran School of Theology in Chicago. A representative of W. K. Kellogg Foundation presented Granger with a citation "for his many contributions to the health and well-being of the American public."

Robert DeVries, program director of the W. K. Kellogg Foundation, said that during his education at the University of Chicago he had also been influenced by Granger, who "sensed suffering beyond that clinically described." DeVries identified five major contributions made by Granger and the people of Wholistic Health Centers.

1. Improved access to and availability of primary medicine.
2. A new, expanded definition of humanism as it applies to medical care.
3. One of the earliest practice forms of what is now called health promotion and heath education.
4. A new definition of the primary care team, with the patient as a full-fledged member.
5. An impact on the church, when many were resigning their role in the health care system.

At the retirement dinner, Joseph Sittler, longtime family friend and "dean of the American theological community," spoke of Granger as being deeply rooted in his theological foundation: "... he has the wonderful advantage of having his principle taproot straight and deep into the heart of the Christian, Hebrew, and Western philosophical tradition ... The soul in Hebrew means the entire person; the fundamental principle ... not a gaseous or effluent liquid."

Sittler also referred to Granger's "sense of the proper moment ... at a time when vehement particularization had struck medicine" and of his "operational methodology; an oleaginous combination which if expressed in other fields would be called seduction. This man can remove your shirt without disturbing your jacket!"

Although the financial model of the Wholistic Health Centers was fraught with challenges, the centers were nevertheless a working laboratory and revealed lasting lessons about health and wellness that informed future efforts by Granger and others.

Rev. G. Scott Morris, MD, the young seminary student who visited the Wholistic Health Center in Hinsdale, Illinois, in the 1970s, drew inspiration from the model for his own vision of ministering to both body and spirit and involving the church in active healing ministries. Church Health in Memphis, Tennessee, which Morris founded, today receives national attention for its model of wellness in both body and spirit and its engagement with the faith, medical, and business communities of Memphis. Dr. Morris's and Church Health's close ties to Granger's legacy have continued to grow, as we will see shortly.

Faith Community Nursing

One of Granger's greatest legacies is the parish nurse movement he began in the 1980s, after becoming convinced of the critical role the nurse plays in health care and health promotion by understanding the whole person. In 2005 the American Nurses Association recognized that as the specialty practice evolved, the term *faith community nursing* would reflect the broad scope of the movement and began to use the new term.[4]

In 1991, the Alexian Brothers and the directors of the Alexian Brothers Medical Center gave their 1992 Modern Samaritan Award to Granger for founding the Wholistic Health Centers and initiating the parish nurse movement that they regarded as designed to integrate the healing ministries of both hospitals and churches.

In 1996, at the tenth annual Westberg Symposium, both Granger and Helen were honored for their contributions to parish nursing. Ann Solari-Twadell and others said that they wanted to be sure to honor Helen because she was the matriarch of the family and the key person in Granger's life. The annual conference now includes separate memorial lectures named for Granger Westberg and Helen Westberg.

The success of the parish nurse movement was even acknowledged in *The Wall Street Journal*. Focusing on some innovations in health care in churches and synagogues, on July 5, 1994 Lewis Andrews wrote:[5]

> In the burgeoning area of outpatient services and aftercare, mainstream religions have created one of the most significant innovations in recent years: the "parish nursing movement." Started in the Midwest almost a decade ago by a Lutheran minister, Granger Westberg, it bases nurses at individual churches and synagogues to meet the health care needs of the congregations.

In 2002, the IPNRC moved to the Deaconess Foundation in St. Louis under the leadership of the Rev. Deborah Patterson. The work of the IPNRC focused on the provision and promotion of education, research and support through curriculum, resources and continuing education opportunities. The IPNRC in St. Louis continued to offer the annual Westberg Symposium, and the lectures that honor Granger and Helen.

In 2011 the IPNRC became part of the Church Health Center in Memphis, Tennessee, bringing together two independent strands of Granger's legacy, a wholistic approach to health care and faith community nursing, in one organization well-positioned to be a key voice in the faith and health values at the heart of Granger's lifelong vision. From its earliest days, faith based nursing has also been a model for Granger's visions of ecumenical programs in the service of healing and wholeness.

Church Health is continuing the annual Westberg Symposia

and regularly updates the *Foundations of Faith Community Nursing* curriculum, which is based on the educational program Granger and his colleagues originally conceived. The curriculum is widely used and available in a variety of formats and settings including weekly classes, online courses, retreat settings, mentoring, and combinations of independent study and class work. About 16,000 nurses across the US and around the world have participated in these courses. Across denominations and faith traditions, every nurse trained in this specialty work practices in the legacy of Granger Westberg.

Faith community nurses practice mainly in the US, but they also practice in close to 30 countries including Australia, the United Kingdom, Korea, Canada, Brazil, Ukraine, and Swaziland. They continue to work in the inner city, the suburbs, and rural areas. The educational attainment of the faith community nurses varies widely, from entry level nursing degrees to doctoral level degrees. Some faith community nurses are paid; others are volunteers. Some work full-time; others work part-time. Some nurses are linked to one or more congregations; some are linked to hospitals or other health care facilities. The faith traditions in which they work include Christian, Jewish, Muslim, Hindu, and Buddhist. Many carry out the roles that Granger identified long ago, such as health educator and educator of volunteers.

Health Ministries Association

The Health Ministries Association continues to fulfill the intent of those who founded the organization after the second Westberg Symposium. Faith community nurses comprise the largest constituency in the organization. The American Nurses Association (ANA) recognizes HMA as the membership organization for this nursing specialty. HMA has continuously championed the work of gaining certification in faith community nursing, including certification by portfolio beginning in 2014. In addition to continued collaboration with the ANA, the American Nurses Credentialing Center, and IPNRC, the Health Ministries Association has formed strong collaborative partnerships with national faith-based and government-based faith-health initiatives and organizations.

In 1996 the Health Ministries Association established the Granger Westberg Lecture Series for providing keynote speakers at the Annual HMA Conferences. Following Granger Westberg's death, HMA planted a tree and had a plaque placed on the campus of Augustana College, Rock Island, Illinois, in honor of Granger's contribution to the faith-health movement. In 2011 HMA established the Granger Westberg Leadership in Faith Community Nursing Award. It recognizes an outstanding faith community nurse who has achieved success in implementing a practice that is faith-centered, community-driven and wholistic in its approach. HMA continues its commitment to awarding this recognition of faith community nurses as part of Granger's ongoing legacy.

Legacies for Generations to Come

For decades, ABC's Dr. Timothy Johnson has been one of America's best known and trusted physicians. When he was a minister in the Evangelical Covenant Church and considering going to medical school, he turned to Granger for guidance. Much later, at Granger's retirement party in 1982, Tim reflected on Granger's influence on his own education and outlined the qualities he said were increasingly being sought by the American public that Granger had anticipated: "communication rather than just commands ... participating rather than just preaching ... caring rather than just curing ... dialogue rather than [being] the object of a diagnosis ... teaching rather than [being] the object of treatment ... insight into prevention rather than just prescriptions ... authority without traditional arrogance."

Granger's influence on his own family is also bringing a continuing impact. Granger sought to influence his own children to pursue some part of his vision. Like many children, Jane, John, Jill, and Joan were initially reluctant to follow their father's path. Yet, his presence is evident in the lives they've shaped for themselves.

Although Jane declined Granger's suggestion that she become a physician, she eventually pursued a doctorate degree focused on medical education, and became a medical school professor. She has worked nationally and internationally for decades with her physician husband, Hilliard Jason, seeking to help enhance the quality of health care by educating collaborative, compassionate physicians who are effective lifelong learners. Now, in what may turn out to be the largest project of their lives, and a natural expression of several of Granger's dreams, they are collaborating in leadership positions in the visioning and planning of a new kind of international, philanthropic medical school.[6]

John carefully shepherds Granger's legacy and estate. John describes himself as having been in the funeral industry for more than 50 years. He operated four Chicagoland cemeteries, and later John and his wife owned a casket company that John started. Through these and many other efforts John helped to give "good grief" to large numbers of people.

Joan, a theater major in college and graduate school, acted in New York and Houston. Later she earned a masters degree in social work from Columbia and worked as a psychiatric social worker in hospital intensive care units, helping those with mental illness transition back into the community.

Jill collaborated with Granger on resources and programs to engage churches in health ministry. She also wrote several books in the field of faith and health,[7] a field in which she continues to work as a consultant. Currently she is living in the cottage on Lake Geneva that her parents built many decades ago. It is steeped in family memories and still is a family gathering place.

As we reflect on Granger's current and future legacy, we have to wonder what students of his students will become the next generation's optimistic, gentle rebels who help make the world a better place for countless others? Probably, Granger's greatest legacy is yet to come.

Q&A with Martin Marty on Granger Westberg

Dr. Martin E. Marty is the one of the world's most prominent scholars of religion and history. As the Fairfax M. Cone Distinguished Service Professor Emeritus at the University of Chicago, he taught for 35 years and is the author of more than 60 books. Yet just as Dr. Marty has been a source of inspiration for thousands of scholars, he too was inspired by fellow scholars and colleagues. One such person was Granger Westberg, an early scholar of the modern pastoral care movement and the founder of parish nursing. He is the subject of the new biography *Gentle Rebel: The Life and Work of Granger Westberg*, and Stacy Smith spoke with Dr. Marty about Granger's life and legacy.

Stacy Smith: Tell me about your history with Granger Westberg, how you met, and how your work intersected.

Martin Marty : I was ordained in 1952 in the Lutheran Church Missouri Synod and served a congregation in River Forest, Illinois as an assistant pastor. I loved parish ministry very much. I had never planned to go for a doctorate, but it was written into the call that the assistant pastor should do doctoral work, so I began that work at the Lutheran School of Theology. Two University of Chicago professors came out and talked to us, and they liked what I was doing and said they would like to give me a free ride to work on a doctorate and teach there. Two years after ordination, I went to the university to study full-time for two years.

Like almost everyone, I came without much background in the things in which Granger Westberg specialized and was an innovator. In seminary we learned how to do bedside prayers and console people and confess people, but there was nothing informatively technical about it. At the university, thanks to Westberg, we were brought into a whole new world and I made a great deal of it. The people with whom he studied—Russell Dicks, for instance—were the founders of the modern pastoral care movement. Westberg became a young scholar at their sides. Before too long after seminary and his own career in pastoral ministry, he was brought to the University of Chicago. He was young and new and always accessible. He ended up with an appointment unique in American theological education, a joint appointment between the medical school and the divinity school.

What are some of your strongest memories of studying with Granger Westberg?

I was not a student in his field, but that made no difference: his influence was widely spread in the Divinity School and the University in general. You'd always know where to find him at lunch—usually one-on-one or one-on-three with medical doctors or other pastoral care people. That was a new thing. He always wore a clerical collar, which not many Protestant pastors did in that day. A doctor once asked him, gruffly, "What are you doing here? We're a med school and we have it all figured out." Westberg said, "What am I doing here? Let's see: everything I do is based on two books, the Hebrew Scriptures and the New Testament. Almost every page talks about people being healed of sickness, leprosy, demonic possession, and other diseases—even guilt. Further, monks, priests, or nuns have always been at the side of the wounded with healing work. They started the first hospital systems. They housed people and hung in there. There was no greater sin for a priest than to skip town when the plague came. Many of them died. Then came the Protestants who trained their married pastors to deal with the families. Now in modern America we think we have to start over, rather than inherit European institutions." Granger paused and said to the physician, "The longer I talk, the more it occurs to me, What are *you* doing here?"

Westberg was not trying be defiant, but it was a teaching venture. He was well read and taught some courses. Many divinity students worked with him.

How would you describe the difference Granger Westberg, a pastor, made in the field of health care?

First, during Westberg's time at the University of Chicago, clinical pastoral education was on the rise, and increasingly students made that their specialty. Granger was a mentor, tutor, and shaper in those fields. He moved on to Texas, but what he built remained. There's a new program at the University of Chicago's medical school that derives in no small measure from Westberg's original impetus. Granger's students carried on, and his curriculum carried on.

Second, Westberg always will be remembered for being the pioneer in supporting a new status and enlarging the role of nurses. When I was at the Park Ridge Center we noticed the nurses were often seen as handmaids to doctors and administrators. Westberg didn't like that. He would say they were colleagues. They needed special recognition and training. My late first wife died from cancer in the clinics there and was ministered to by nurses who benefited from Westberg's innovations and legacies. By then the nurses had gotten their charter from Westberg, and they said they didn't feel inferior.

A Canadian scholar wrote a book about *The Renewal of Generosity: Health, Illness, and How to Live*. When I urged my second wife to read it, she asked me why. I said, "There is one sentence, and if it doesn't persuade you to read it, nothing will. It's very Westbergian."

The author quoted a woman who said, "My doctor cured me, but she didn't heal me; she never once looked in my face."

Westberg recognized the importance of pulling up a chair, sitting down, looking the patient in the face and saying, "Please tell me your story." In ten minutes patients would impart things that enabled the physician to be more helpful than would have been possible with only the results of tests and exams. This focus on listening to patients is what is, in part, behind the founding of the parish nurse program, which is now huge. I got to speak at the first annual Westberg Symposium in 1987. There wasn't enough space for all the people who came already back then.

You used the term *Westbergian*. What would you say is the essence of *Westbergiana*?

Face-to-face, listening, encouraging the other, lifelong learning, making connections.

It's not hard to get your name in print and win prizes if you're the head of a medical school or make some discovery. Westberg's hard to pin down because everything he did was relational. Because he excelled in several fields, and he focused on enabling others, Westberg's profile is less clear than that of some in parallel disciplines. But I'd like it if he is enduringly seen as a founder of the new status for the chaplain, pastor, and spiritual counselor, in the bedside clinic and in the lab.

What do you think would have excited Granger Westberg about a new focus on health care in the US, and what would be his frustration?

I think the two would come together. What excited him was the challenge of overcoming what frustrated him. The technology of medicine can reduce everything to a pattern of efficiency. Sherwin Nuland wrote the book *How We Die*. We became friends. One year, when he was to speak at Northwestern's Medical School graduation, my wife invited him and his wife over for breakfast beforehand. I asked him, "What are you going to tell the new MDs?" He said, "I'm going to tell them you can never know too much science to be a good physician, and you can never forget enough science to be good at the bedside." And that's very close to what this is about. How do you humanize the wonders of technology?

Westberg would say the gains also brought losses. In some ways America is both more religious and more secular. It is more religious in that more people turn to everything from alternative medicine, Chinese medicine, New Age remedies, and all this has religious tinges. And of course there is still the Judeo-Christian mindset. But we're also more secular in that more health decisions are made without any transcendent order. I think Westberg would accept the challenge of bridging that divide.

This article was written by Stacy Smith for the Spring 2015 issue of Church Health Reader. *For more information visit, chreader.org.*

Chronology of the Life and Work of Granger Westberg

1913   Granger's birth

1935   Enters Augustana Theological Seminary

1939   Ordination into Augustana Lutheran Church
Marriage to Helen Johnson
Pastor of First English Lutheran Church (now St. John's
Lutheran Church) in Bloomington, Illinois

1944   Chaplain of Augustana Lutheran Hospital

1946   Chaplain of the newly organized Association of Protestant
Hospital Chaplains

1952   Chaplain of the University of Chicago Clinics. Associate
professor of pastoral care in the Federated Theology Faculty

1956   Professor of religion and health, University of Chicago; joint
appointment in the schools of medicine and theology

1964   Dean of the Institute of Religion (now the Institute of Religion
and Health). Professor of medicine and religion in the
department of psychiatry of Baylor University College of
Medicine.

1967   Professor of practical theology and continuing education at
        Hamma School of Theology, Wittenberg University, in
        Springfield, Ohio

1968   Grant to establish the Academy of Parish Clergy

1970   Opening of first Church Clinic

1973   Professor of preventive medicine, University of Illinois School
        of Medicine
        First Wholistic Health Center opened in Hinsdale, Illinois

1983   Pilot program for Parish Nurse Project in Tucson, Arizona

1985   With the support and collaboration of Lutheran General
        Hospital parish nurses began work in six churches

1986   Parish Nurse Resource Center

1987   First Granger Westberg Parish Nurse Symposium

1989   Health Ministries Association formed

1996   Health Ministries Association established the Granger
        Westberg lecture series

1999   Death of Granger Westberg

Acknowledgments

I began writing this book a year before Dad died, more than 16 years ago. Thankfully, he had kept scrapbooks, articles, papers, and photos of his life and career that were helpful to us as Dad and I pieced together his history. Even though Parkinson's disease made it difficult for him to talk, he recounted many stories that I recorded and transcribed and included in this book.

A couple of times after Dad's death, I tried to pull the book together. My sisters, Jill Westberg McNamara and Joan Westberg Onder, patiently critiqued and added to what I had written. I gathered more stories from our mother, Helen Johnson Westberg; our brother, John Westberg; and key people who had worked with Dad. However, my professional work made it difficult for me to give the manuscript the attention it needed.

The manuscript, which grew thick over the years, would have remained on a shelf had it not been for Jill's encouragement and support, and her help with the manuscript. I'm grateful also for her perspective as the youngest child in the family. We are 13 years apart in age, so I have firsthand memories of Dad's early career, while Jill has memories of working with Dad in the days of the Wholistic Health Centers and the beginning of the parish nurse movement. I gave some help to Dad when he wrote *Minister and Doctor Meet*. Many years later, Jill helped Dad with several books.

The completion of this book is also thanks to our sister, Joan; my husband, Hilliard (Hill) Jason; and our editor, Susan Martins Miller, who was a great help in trimming and organizing the manuscript. We are also grateful for the contributions of other members of the Church Health staff, especially John Shorb, who helped get the project off the ground, Stacy Smith, who shepherded the project, and Lizy Heard, who designed the book's layout. Also we appreciate Bill Maloney and Todd Hochberg's resourcefulness in finding some photos from Dad's days at Lutheran General Hospital.

Notes

Chapter 1: Only the Beginning

1. Granger Westberg, "Why Me, Lord," *The Disciple* 13, no. 9, May 21, 1985, 20–22. Granger Westberg, "Why Me, Lord." *The Lutheran* (September 1986): 5–6.
2. The name "Augustana" was drawn from the Augsburg Confession that was created in 1530 during the time of the Reformation.
3. This is the first of many quotations in the text that came from my recorded conversations with Granger (Dad).

Chapter 2: Fast Talking

1. Granger Westberg, "Are Ministers in a Rut?" *Augustana Seminary Review* 11 no. 2 (1959): 20–24
2. Granger Westberg, "Are Ministers in a Rut?" 20.
3. In 1970, Elizabeth Platz, a graduate of Gettysburg Seminary, became the first female Lutheran pastor in North America.

Chapter 3: The Larger Vision

1. George M. Stephenson, *The Religious Aspects of Swedish Immigration* (Minneapolis: University of Minnesota Press, June 1932).
2. Playing the piano in keys with multiple sharps or flats is typically more challenging for pianists than playing pieces written in keys with only one or two sharps or flats.
3. Granger Westberg, "The Art of Worship," *The Lutheran Companion*, May 30, 1936, 684–685. The other three articles in *The Lutheran Companion* series are "Three Important Rooms," "The Altar," and "The Morning Service."
4. Granger Westberg, "The Risk of Openness," *The Hamma Bulletin*, January 1969, 7.
5. C. A. Wendell, *The Larger Vision: A Study of the Evolution Theory in its Relation to the Christian Faith* (Minneapolis, MN: Self-published, 1925).
6. Granger Westberg, "The Risk of Openness," *The Hamma Bulletin*, January 1969, 7.
7. G. Everett Arden, *The School of the Prophets: The Background and History*

of Augustana Theological Seminary, 1860-1960 (Rock Island, IL: Augustana Theological Seminary, 1960), 233.

8. Richard Cabot and Russell Dicks, *The Art of Ministering to the Sick* (New York: Macmillan, 1936).

9. Russell L. Dicks, "The Art of Ministering to the Sick," *Pastoral Psychology*, November 1952, 10.

Chapter 4: Ringing Church Bells

1. Petrus Olaf Bersell was the president of the Augustana Church from 1935-1951.

2. $1,000 in 1940 was the equivalent of $16,646.35 in 2014.

3. Granger Westberg, "The Church as 'Health Place,'" *Dialog: A Journal of Theology* 27, no. 2 (Winter, 1988): 189-195.

4. Granger Westberg, "Marry Us, Reverend," *The Lutheran Companion*, July 31, 1941. Reprinted in *Religious Digest* (September, 1941): 50-52.

5. Granger Westberg, "Are Church Hospitals Different?" *The Augustana Quarterly* 12, no. 1 (January 1943): 53-63.

6. Granger Westberg, "Have You Ever Tried Counseling?" The *Lutheran Outlook*, September 1944. Reprinted in Religious Digest, Grand Rapids, MI: William B. Eerdmans Publishing Company (November 1944): 71-74.

7. Granger Westberg, "Have You Ever Tried Counseling?" *The Lutheran Outlook*, September 1944.

Chapter 5: Thrown to the Wolves

1. Granger Westberg, *Minister and Doctor Meet* (New York: Harper and Row, 1961), 3.

2. Granger Westberg, *Minister and Doctor Meet*, (New York: Harper and Row, 1961), 6.

3. Granger Westberg, "Are Church Hospitals Different?" *The Augustana Quarterly* 12, no. 1 (January 1943): 53-63.

4. Granger Westberg, "Pioneering in Church Hospitals," *The Lutheran Outlook*, May 1943, 80-82.

Chapter 6: Verbatim

1. Kirsten Peachey and Charles D. Phillips, "The College of Chaplains: The First 25 Years," *The Caregiver Journal* 12, no. 1 (1996): 6-17.

2. Russell L. Dicks, "The Hospital Chaplain," *Pastoral Psychology* (April 1950): 50-54.

3. O. V. Anderson, letter to Granger Westberg, September 23, 1943.

4. Russell L. Dicks, letter to Granger Westberg, September 29, 1943.

5. Anton Boisen, *Exploration of the Inner Life: A Study of Mental Disorder and Religious Experience* (Philadelphia: University of Pennsylvania, 1971).

6. Edward E. Thorton, *Professional Education for Ministry: A History of Clinical Pastoral Education* (Nashville: Abingdon Press, 1970), 102.

7. John Evans, "New Chaplain's Plan Tried in Hospital Here." [newspaper article; no identifying information]

8. V. J. Tengwald, "A Unique Church Mission," *The Lutheran Companion* (1941) 2-3.

9. Helen K. Grace, "Nursing." In *Handbook of Health Professions Education*, ed.

Christine H. McGuire, Richard Foley, Alan Gorr, Ronald W. Richards et al. (San Francisco: Jossey-Bass Publishers, 1983), 92–112. According to Grace, nursing was regarded as a good preparation for marriage.

10. W. C. Alvarez, "Spiritual Help Aids Physical Ills," *Los Angeles Times*, October 6, 1958. Also (October 19, 1958) same article appeared in "Keeping Well" column with heading "How Ministers Can Help the Ill."

11. Erich Lindemann, "Symptomatology and the Management of Acute Grief," *The American Journal of Psychiatry* 101 (September 1944): 141–148.

12. Granger Westberg, "What a Congregation Looks Like that Takes Wholistic Health Seriously," in *Health Care and Its Costs: A Challenge for the Church*, ed. Walter E. Wiest, (Lantham, New York, and London: University Press of America, 1988).

13. Granger Westberg. "The Interrelationship of the Ministry and Medicine." *Pastoral Psychology*, April, 1957, 9–13.

14. Granger Westberg, "Will They Be Happy? A Guide to Marriage," *The Lutheran Companion*, February 2, 1949, 6–7.

15. Granger Westberg, "The Hospital Chaplain," manuscript sent to Vergilius Ferm April, 1954.

16. In this era, most nursing schools were linked to hospitals, not to colleges or universities.

17. Granger Westberg, *Nurse, Pastor, and Patient* (Rock Island, IL: Augustana Book Concern, 1955).

Chapter 7: Whet the Appetite

1. Granger Westberg, "A Seminar in a Hospital," *The Lutheran Companion*, August 1945, 8–9.

2. Granger Westberg, "A Seminar in a Hospital," *The Lutheran Companion*, August 1945, 8–9.

3. Helen Fleming, "Clergymen Talk Too Much, Seminar on Counseling Told," *The Chicago Daily News*, July 10, 1951.

4. Brief History of the US Army Chaplaincy Corp http://www.usachcs.army.mil/history/brief/chapter_6.htm

5. E. Brooks Holifield, *A History of Pastoral Care in America: From Salvation to Self-Realization* (Nashville: Abingdon Press, 1983), 269–70.

6. Others in attendance included John Billinsky, Carl R. Plack, John R. Thomas, Robert Morris, Leicester Potter, and Carl Scherzer.

7. Julian Byrd and Arne K. Jessen, "The College of Chaplains of the American Protestant Health Association," *Journal of Pastoral Care* 42 no. 3 (Fall, 1988): 228–30.

8. Granger Westberg, "A New Vision of the Chaplain of Tomorrow from a Personal Friend of Russell Dicks," Russell L. Dicks Memorial Lecture, 1990.

9. Edgar Blake, a trained hospital administrator. Personal communication between John Thomas and Jane Westberg.

10. Although Dicks's work in Chicago was short-lived, he went on to have a

distinguished career. From 1948 until 1958 he was professor of pastoral care at the Divinity School of Duke University and ex officio chaplain of the Duke University Hospital from 1948 to 1956. Dicks was a prolific writer and a popular lecturer. He was editor of *Religion and Health*, a journal to which Granger made numerous contributions.

11. Granger Westberg, "An Organized Chaplaincy Service," Unpublished manuscript, 1947.

12. Granger Westberg, "Sermon Preached in a Hospital Chapel." Unpublished manuscript, probably written in the mid-1950s because Granger is listed as professor of religion and health.

13. Granger Westberg, "So You're a Family Man," Lincolnwood PTA, 1948. [Handwritten notes.]

14. Granger Westberg's handwritten notes with no title.

15. Hiltner had served as secretary under Helen Dunbar at the Council of Clinical Training for Theological Students from 1935 to 1938.

16. Seward Hiltner, *Pastoral Counseling* (Nashville, Tennessee: Abingdon Press, 1949). He had already written *Religion and Health* (New York: Macmillan Company, 1943).

17. "Man of the Month: Seward Hiltner," *Pastoral Psychology* 2, no. 13 (April 15, 1951): 1, 65.

18. E. Brooks Holifield claimed that the publication of Carl Rogers's book, *Counseling and Psychotherapy* (Boston: Houghton Mifflin Company, 1942) created hardly a ripple among academic psychologists, but it quickly became a standard text in seminaries. E. Brooks Holifield. *A History of Pastoral Care in America: From Salvation to Self-Realization.* (Nashville: Abingdon Press, 1983), 295.

19. Carl Rogers wrote: "Psychologists and psychiatrists need to do more profound thinking about the problem of values, which is so deeply involved in all of their work. Here the thinking of the minister and theologian should be of help." Carl Rogers, "Through the Eyes of the Client," *Pastoral Psychology* 1, no. 2 (March 1950): 66.

Chapter 8: Walls Built So High

1. Prior to Granger's arrival at the university, a part-time "traveling" Lutheran chaplain had provided some services.

2. The four seminaries, which had been on the Chicago campus when Lael began working there in the early 1930s, joined in a cooperative endeavor called the Federated Theological Faculty (FTF). The FTF was based in the Chicago Divinity School but had close ties with Chicago Theological Seminary, Disciples Divinity House, and the Meadville Theological School. Members of the Federated Theology Faculty worked closely together and offered many courses in common. In 1960 the joint venture was discontinued, but the faculties continued working together in a less formal way.

3. The hospitals included the Albert Merritt Billings (a general hospital); Max Epstein Clinic; Bob Roberts Memorial Hospital for Children; and the Chicago

Lying-in Hospital (a maternity hospital).

4. *Journal of Medical Education*, January 1954.

5. Granger Westberg, "The Chaplain in the Modern Hospital," *The Bulletin of Maternal Welfare*, March/April, 1954, 11–13.

6. Granger Westberg, "The Chaplain in the Modern Hospital," *The Bulletin of Maternal Welfare*, March/April 1954, 11–13.

7. Granger Westberg, "The 'New' Field of Religion and Medicine," *Postgraduate Medicine* 23, no. 6 (1958): 668.

8. Seward Hiltner, "Man of the Month: Granger Westberg," *Pastoral Psychology*, August 1955, 6, 66.

9. Granger Westberg, "The Interrelationship of the Ministry and Medicine," *Pastoral Psychology*, April 1957, 9–13.

10. Granger Westberg, "Interrelationship of the Ministry and Medicine," *Pastoral Psychology*, April 1957, 9–13, 55.

11. For example, a letter from Rabbi Eric Friedland indicated that Granger had spoken to his congregation in 1957 and was going to do so again in 1958.

12. Granger Westberg, "Ministering to the Sick," *Central Conference American Rabbis* 2 (1953): 28–33.

13. Asclepius was the Greek god of healing. People believed they could be cured in temples dedicated to Asclepion. People were cared for by priest healers called the Asclepiadae.

14. Ta-Nehisi Coates, "The Case for Reparations," *The Atlantic*, June 2014. http://www.theatlantic.com/features/archive/2014/05/the-case-for-reparations/361631/

15. In 1517 as part of his mission to reform the Roman Catholic Church, Martin Luther King, a friar, Catholic priest, and theologian, nailed 95 theses to the door of the church in Wittenberg.

16. List of Advisory Board Members. *Pastoral Psychology*, February 1954, 10.

17. Granger Westberg, "A Next Step in Ecumenicity," Sermon at Rockefeller Memorial Chapel, February 27, 1955.

18. Granger and his Lutheran colleagues were promised the land in exchange for the land on which Augustana Church, the Westberg family's church, then stood.

19. Augustana Evangelical Lutheran Church of Swedish background, the Association of Evangelical Lutheran Churches of Danish background, and the Suomi Synod (Finish Evangelical Lutheran Church of America).

20. (1) Granger Westberg, "The Cancer Patient and His Spiritual Needs. April 1954 Manuscript. (2) Granger Westberg, "The Spiritual Needs of the Patient,"(Comments also by John J. Flanagan, SJ and Rabbi Samuel M. Silver). *Parish Nurse Digest* 30, no. 3 (September, 1955): 16. (3) Granger Westberg, "The Nurse is the Chaplain's Ally," *The Modern Hospital* 84, no. 4 (April, 1955): 82, 137; (4) Granger Westberg, "The Hospital Chaplain," manuscript sent to Vergilius Ferm April 1954.

21. Granger Westberg, *Nurse, Pastor, and Patient: A Hospital Chaplain Talks to Nurses* (Rock Island, IL: Augustana Book Concern, 1955).

22. Granger Westberg, *Nurse, Pastor, and Patient: A Hospital Chaplain Talks to Nurses* (Rock Island, IL: Augustana Book Concern, 1955).

Chapter 9: A Pioneering Joint Appointment

1. *Time Magazine*, April 16, 1956, 55.
2. *Pastoral Psychology*, June 1956, 62.
3. Granger Westberg, "Religious Aspects of Medical Teaching," *Journal of Medical Education* 32 no. 3 (March 1957): 204-209.
4. "The Whole Patient: Synthesis of Medicine, Religion," *AMA News*, April 20, 1959, 3.
5. Granger Westberg, *Minister and Doctor Meet* (New York: Harper and Row, 1961), 82.
6. From a 1983 article on Granger and his work in the University of Arizona's campus newspaper, *InforMed*.
7. Granger Westberg, "From Hospital Chaplaincy to Wholistic Health Center," *The Journal of Pastoral Care* 33, no. 2 (1979): 76-82.
8. Granger Westberg, "From Hospital Chaplaincy to Wholistic Health Center," *The Journal of Pastoral Care* 33, no. 2 (1979): 76-82.
9. Granger Westberg, "The Interrelationship of the Ministry and Medicine," *Pastoral Psychology* (April 1957): 9-13.
10. Granger Westberg, *Sjuksköterskan, Prästen och Patienten*, trans. Brita and Bertil Werkström (Stockholm: Diakonistyr, 1962).

Chapter 10: Working and Learning in Communities

1. Granger Westberg, "The Interrelationship of the Ministry and Medicine," *Pastoral Psychology*, April 1957, 9-13.
2. *Pastoral Psychology*. April, 1957, p. 55.
3. Granger Westberg, "The Role of the Clergyman in Mental Health," *Pastoral Psychology*, May 1960, 19-22.
4. Faculty from the school of divinity included Seward Hiltner, Alvin Pitcher, and Joseph Sittler. Faculty from the medicine school included Joseph Evans, Joseph Kirsner, Cornelius Vermeulen, Henry Wildberger, C. Knight Aldrich, and Robert S. Daniels.
5. Granger Westberg, "The Role of the Clergyman in Mental Health," *Pastoral Psychology*, May 1960, 19-22.
6. Granger Westberg, "Parish Clergymen and Mental Health: The Kokomo and La Grange Projects." Chapter 28 in Howard J. Clinebell, *Community Mental Health—the Role of Church and Temple* (New York, Abingdon Press, 1970). <www.religion-online.org/showchapter.asp?title=798&C=1025>
7. Austin Wehrwein, "Clergy Briefed on Mental Ills," *The New York Times*, January 11, 1959.
8. Granger Westberg and Edgar Draper, *Community Psychiatry and the Clergyman* (Springfield, IL: Charles C. Thomas, 1966).
9. Granger Westberg, "Parish Clergymen and Mental Health: The Kokomo and La Grange Projects." Chapter 28 in Howard J. Clinebell, *Community Mental Health— the Role of Church and Temple* (New York: Abingdon Press 1970). <www.religion-online.org/showchapter.asp?title=798&C=1025>

10. Granger Westberg and Edgar Draper, *Community Psychiatry and the Clergyman* (Springfield, IL: Charles C. Thomas, 1966).

11. Hans Hofman, ed., *The Ministry and Mental Health* (New York: Association Press, 1960).

12. Granger Westberg, "The Need for Radical Changes in Theological Education: A Proposed 44-Month Plan." In *The Ministry and Mental Health*, ed. Hans Hofman (New York: Association Press, 1960), 167–182.

13. Granger Westberg, "The Need for Radical Changes," In *The Ministry and Mental Health*, ed. Hans Hofman (New York: Association Press, 1960), 167.

14. Granger Westberg, "Avenues to Health through Religion," [Manuscript with no identification except that Granger was an associate professor of religion and health, so he would have written it in the period 1956–1962.]

15. Granger Westberg, "The Pastor Reassesses His Role in Preventive Psychiatry." [Talk given in 1962 or 1963.]

16. Seward Hiltner, "Review of *Minister and Doctor Meet*," *The Journal of Religion* (1961): 300. Hiltner sent a copy of his review to Granger with his note: "Granger: this is for the J of Rel. Hope you like it. It is a good book. Seward."

17. Orville S. Walters, "Psychiatry and Clergyman. Review of *Minister and Doctor Meet*," November 10, 1961. [No further identifying information on clipping.]

18. Wayne Oates. Review of *Minister and Doctor Meet. Pastoral Psychology*, June 1961, 55–56.

Chapter 11: Good Grief

1. Erich Lindemann, "Symptomatology and the Management of Acute Grief," *The American Journal of Psychiatry* 101 (September, 1944): 141–148. (Lindemann described five stages he observed in the acute grief process: (1) somatic distress; (2) preoccupation with the image of the deceased; (3) guilt; (4) hostile reactions; and (5) loss of patterns of conduct).

2. Granger Westberg, *Good Grief* (Philadelphia: Fortress Press, 1962).

3. Charles M. Schultz, *Good Grief*, Charlie Brown (Robinsdale, MN: Fawcett Publication, 1963).

4. Granger Westberg, *Good Grief* (Philadelphia: Fortress Press, 1962).

5. A. Einar Farstrug of the American Evangelical Lutheran Church; Malvin H. Lundeen of the Augustana Lutheran Church; Raymond Wargelin of the Suomi Synod; and Franklin Clark Fry of the United Lutheran Church

6. G. Everett Arden, *Augustana Heritage: A History of the Augustana Lutheran Church* (Rock Island, IL: Augustana Press, 1963), 411–412.

7. Augustana Seminary (Augustana Evangelical Lutheran Church); Maywood Seminary (United Lutheran Church in America); Suomi Seminary (Finnish Evangelical Lutheran Church); and Grand View Seminary (American Evangelical Lutheran Church).

8. Neil Jillett, two articles under "News of the Day" titled "Agnostic" and "Black Shirt." Melborne newspaper, August 22, 1963.

Chapter 12: Raising the Curtain on Three Acts of Illness

1. Granger Westberg, "Expansion Opportunities for the Office of Medicine and Religion," unpublished manuscript, December 19–20, 1963.
2. Granger Westberg, "The Challenge of the Hospital Chaplaincy—1964," Opening address of Special Invitation Conference on Hospital Chaplaincy. Sponsored by the American Medical Association and the American Hospital Association, 1964.
3. Granger Westberg, "The Challenge of the Hospital Chaplaincy—1964," Opening address of Special Invitation Conference on Hospital Chaplaincy. Sponsored by the American Medical Association and the American Hospital Association, 1964.
4. Granger Westberg, "The Three Acts of Illness," *Christian Living*, February 1967, 8–10.
5. Letter from Stanley Bennett to Granger Westberg, July 16, 1964.
6. *Pastoral Psychology*, June 1964, 56.

Chapter 13: The Living Human Document

1. E. E. Thornton, *Professional Education for Ministry: A History of Clinical Pastoral Education* (Nashville: Abingdon Press, 1970), 148.
2. The five seminaries, which used the Institute as a "laboratory extension," were Austin Presbyterian Theological Seminary in Austin; Brite Divinity School (Disciples of Christ) at Texas Christian University in Fort Worth; Episcopal Theological Seminary of the Southwest in Austin; Perkins School of Theology at Southern Methodist University in Dallas; and Southwestern Baptist Theological Seminary in Fort Worth. Students were also accepted at the Institute from other schools.
3. Brochure of the Institute of Religion.
4. Methodist Hospital is a major teaching hospital located next to the Institute of Religion.
5. Dr. Michael DeBakey was a world famous cardiovascular surgeon.
6. Robert Graham Kemper, "Granger Westberg on Pastoral Care," *The Christian Ministry* 3, no. 4 (July 1972): 15–17, 42–44.
7. Mary Merryfield, "Everybody Grieves at Some Time or Other," *Chicago Tribune*, March 20, 1965.
8. Personal communication between Julian Byrd and Jane Westberg,1998.
9. Granger Westberg, "New Directions in Theological Education." [February 1971 manuscript; no other identification given.]
10. Granger Westberg, "New Directions in Theological Education." [February 1971 manuscript; no other identification given.]
11. Granger Westberg, "Churches Are Joining the Health Care Team," *Urban Health*, October 1984, 34–36.

Chapter 14: The Minister's Finest Hour

1. Granger Westberg, "The Risk of Openness. *The Hamma Bulletin* 7, no. 1 (January 1969): 7.
2. Granger Westberg, "New Directions in Theological Education" (February, 1971).

3. Carl T. Uehling, "Ohio: A New Style Seminary," *The Lutheran*, June 18, 1969, 5–9.

4. Granger Westberg, "The Parish Pastor's Finest Hour," February 26, 1968. Talk given at installation of a pastor.

5. Granger Westberg, "Health, Healing and Salvation: The Health Situation in America Today." [1969 convocation lectures.]

6. "Grant Made for Proposed Clergy Educational Group," *The Lutheran*, 1968, 34.

7. Granger Westberg, "An American Academy of Parish Clergy: Why Not?" *The Christian Century*, April 28, 1965.

8. Besides Granger, other members of the original board were Henry Adams, George Davis, F. Dean Lueking, Richard Mueller, James B. Pierce, Glen O. Peterman, Ralph E. Peterson, and James P. Roach.

9. Granger Westberg, "An Academy for Parish Clergy. *The Hamma Bulletin* 7, no. 3 (1969): 20–21.

10. "Academy of Parish Clergy Founded," *The Christian Century* (1969): 704.

11. http://www.apclergy.org/ourhistory.html

Chapter 15: Creating a Church Clinic

1. Paul Starr, *The Social Transformation of American Medicine* (New York: Basic Books, Inc., 1982), 382.

2. Granger Westberg, "The Church Should Reenter the Health Field: A Proposal for Neighborhood Church-Clinics and a New Medical Specialist—The Clergy Physician." [convocation address, 1969]

3. Granger Westberg, "The Church Should Reenter the Health Field: A Proposal for Neighborhood Church-Clinics and a New Medical Specialist—The Clergy-Physician." [convocation address, 1969]

4. Granger Westberg, "From Hospital Chaplaincy to Wholistic Health Center," *The Journal of Pastoral Care* 33, no. 2 (June 1979): 76–82.

5. Granger Westberg, Progress Report to the Kellogg Foundation, September, 1971.

6. The churches that co-sponsored the project were Clifton Avenue Methodist, St. Joseph Roman Catholic, and Trinity African Methodist.

7. Donald A. Tubesing, *Whole Person Health Care, An Idea in Evolution: History of the Wholistic Health Centers Project 1970-1976* (Chicago: Wholistic Health Centers Inc., 1976), 5.

8. Granger Westberg, *How to Start a Church-Based Clinic*, Charles F. Kettering Foundation, 1975. Also progress report on church-clinical project, May 1970.

9. Granger Westberg, "Dissemination of Wholistic Health Centers," July 17, 1978. [This paper became a chapter in a Kellogg report about dissemination.]

10. Jon L Joyce, "Healing Body and Spirit," *The Lutheran*, March 3, 1971, 12–14.

11. Granger Westberg, "Thoughts on Teaching of Pastoral Care." [unpublished manuscript]

12. Granger Westberg, Progress Report: Neighborhood Church Clinic, September, 1971.

13. Donald A. Tubesing, *Whole Person Health Care, An Idea in Evolution: History of the Wholistic Health Centers Project 1970-1976* (Chicago: Wholistic Health

Centers Inc., 1976), 11.

14. "Clergymen Hear a New Calling: in Doctor's Office," *The National Observer*, December 4, 1971.

15. Paul C. Holinger and Granger E. Westberg, "The Parish Pastor's Finest Hour—Revisited," *Journal of Religion and Health* 14, no. 1 (1975): 14–19.

16. Granger Westberg, "From Hospital Chaplaincy to Wholistic Health Center," *The Journal of Pastoral Care* 33, no. 2 (1979): 76–82.

17. Granger Westberg, *How to Start a Church-based Clinic*, 1975.

18. Granger Westberg, "Contextual Teaching of Pastoral Care in a Neighborhood Church Clinic," in *Explorations in Ministry: A Report on the Ministry in the 70's Project*, ed. Louis Douglass (New York: IDOC-North America 1971): 174–190.

19. Granger Westberg, "Contextual Teaching of Pastoral Care in a Neighborhood Church Clinic," in *Explorations in Ministry: A Report on the Ministry in the 70's Project*, ed. Louis Douglass. (New York: IDOC-North America 1971): 174–190.

Chapter 16: A 30-Year Dream

1. Donald A. Tubesing, *Whole Person Health Care, An Idea in Evolution: History of the Wholistic Health Centers Project 1970-1976* (Chicago: Wholistic Health Centers Inc., 1976), 19.

2. Granger Westberg, "Dissemination of Wholistic Health Centers," Report for Kellogg Foundation, 1973.

3. Donald A. Tubesing, *Whole Person Health Care, An Idea in Evolution: History of the Wholistic Health Centers Project 1970-1976* (Chicago: Wholistic Health Centers Inc., 1976), 28–29.

4. Donald A. Tubesing, *Whole Person Health Care, An Idea in Evolution: History of the Wholistic Health Centers Project 1970-1976* (Chicago: Wholistic Health Centers Inc., 1976), 27.

Chapter 17: As a Matter of Faith

1. Donald A. Tubesing, *Whole Person Health Care, An Idea in Evolution: History of the Wholistic Health Centers Project 1970-1976* (Chicago: Wholistic Health Centers Inc., 1976), 39.

2. Robert Cunningham, *The Wholistic Health Centers: A New Direction in Health Care* (Battle Creek, MI, W.K. Kellogg Foundation, 1977).

3. Donald Tubesing, Paul C. Holinger, Granger E. Westberg, and Edward A. Lichter, "The Wholistic Health Center Project: An Action-Research Model for Providing Preventive, Whole-Person Health Care at the Primary Level," *Medical Care* 15, no. 3 (1977): 217.

4. Jill Westberg, "Hope," in *Theological Roots of Wholistic Health Care: A Response to the Religious Questions that Have Been Raised*, ed. Granger Westberg (Hinsdale, IL: Wholistic Health Center, Inc., 1979), 73–92.

Chapter 18: Life Is a Leaky Boat

1. Granger Westberg, "Case Statement and Development," *Wholistic Wellspring*, Summer 1982, 9–10.
2. Ann Solari-Twadell pointed out that when Granger made this statement, he apparently was not aware of the American Nurses Association's important role in national policy development. E-mail from Ann Solari-Twadell to Jane Westberg, January 3, 2015.
3. Interview of John Riedel by Jane Westberg, 1997.

Chapter 19: Retirement or Refirement?

1. The nine WHCS reported earlier in 1981 were the WHC of Hinsdale, the WHC of Woodridge, the WHC of Mendota, Circle Christian Health Center (originally Austin-Chicago); the WHC of Oak Park, the WHC of La Grange, and the WHC of Oak Lawn. Outside of Chicago there were two WHCs: Trinity Health Care in Minneapolis and Columbia Road Health Services in Washington, DC. *Wholistic Wellspring*, Fall 1981, 12.
2. Bruce Buursma, "Wholistic Centers Heal Spiritually," *The Chicago Tribune*, November 13, 1981.
3. Personal handwritten papers.
4. "A Year of Challenge, Wholistic Health Centers, Inc." Annual Report to W. K. Kellogg Foundation, 1981.

Chapter 20: Nurse in the Church

1. Bruce Buursma, "Pastor Crusades for 'Nurses in Churches,' *The Chicago Tribune*, August 21, 1983
2. Letter to Kent E. Eklund at Lutheran Brotherhood from Granger Westberg, July 7, 1983. The letter refers to earlier communications that indicate Granger had formed these ideas earlier.
3. Helen Grace, PhD, formerly dean of the University of Illinois School of Nursing, joined the W. K. Kellogg Foundation, as vice president for program. Later, still at Kellogg, she became special assistant to the president.
4. Floramae Geiser, "Clinic in a Choir Room," *The Lutheran*, December 1985, 15–16.

Chapter 21: Flight Test

1. *Beginnings ... Perspectives on Parish Nursing, Then and Now* (1997). A videotape produced by Advocate Health Care for the International Parish Nurse Resource Center.
2. *Beginnings ... Perspectives on Parish Nursing, Then and Now* (1997). A videotape produced by Advocate Health Care for the International Parish Nurse Resource Center.
3. Granger Westberg with Jill Westberg, *The Parish Nurse: How to Start a Parish Nurse Program in Your Church* (Park Ridge, IL: Parish Nurse Resource Center (1987), 7.
4. Granger Westberg with Jill Westberg, *The Parish Nurse: How to Start a Parish*

Nurse Program in Your Church (Park Ridge, Illinois: Parish Nurse Resource Center (1987), 9.

5. *Beginnings ... Perspectives on Parish Nursing, Then and Now* (1997). A videotape produced by Advocate Health Care for the International Parish Nurse Resource Center.

6. Lawrence E. Holst, "The Parish Nurse," *Chronicle of Pastoral Care* 7, no. 1 (Spring/Summer 1987): 13–17.

7. Granger Westberg with Jill Westberg, *The Parish Nurse: How to Start a Parish Nurse Program in Your Church* (Park Ridge, L: Parish Nurse Resource Center, 1987).

8. Granger Westberg with Jill Westberg, *The Parish Nurse: How to Start a Parish Nurse Program in Your Church* (Park Ridge, IL: Parish Nurse Resource Center, 1987). 331–32.

9. Granger Westberg with Jill Westberg, *The Parish Nurse: How to Start a Parish Nurse Program in Your Church* (Park Ridge, IL: Parish Nurse Resource Center, 1987).

10. *Beginnings ... Perspectives on Parish Nursing, Then and Now* (1997). A videotape produced by Advocate Health Care for the International Parish Nurse Resource Center.

Chapter 22: Johnny Appleseed of Parish Nursing

1. Granger Westberg with Jill Westberg, *The Parish Nurse: How to Start a Parish Nurse Program in Your Church* (Park Ridge, IL: Parish Nurse Resource Center, 1987).

2. Personal communication by e-mail between Judith Ryan and Jane Westberg, May 19, 1997.

Chapter 23: Traveling on a Single Track

1. Granger Westberg with Jill Westberg McNamara, *The Parish Nurse: Providing a Minister of Health for Your Congregation* (Minneapolis: Augsburg, 1990), 11.

2. For descriptions of different models of faith community nursing see Alexander Rödlach "Faith Community Nursing: An Emerging Ministry of Health and Healing with the Church," *Verbum* 54, no. 2 (2013): 139–165.

3. Ann Solari-Twadell, Mary Ann McDermott, Judith Ryan, and Anne Marie Djupe, *Assuring Visibility for the Future: Guideline Development for Parish Nurse Education Programs*. Park Ridge, IL: Lutheran General Health System, 1994.

4. Mary Ann McDermott, Phyllis Ann Solari-Twadell and R Matheus, "Promoting Quality Education for the Parish Nurse and the Parish Nurse Coordinator," *Nursing and Health Care Perspective* 19, no. 1 (January/February 1998): 4–6.

5. American Nursing Association and Health Ministries Association, *Scope and Standards of Practice: Faith Community Nursing*, 2nd ed. (Silver Springs, MD: American Nurses Association, 2012).

6. P. Ann Solari-Twadell, Anne Marie Djupe, eds. *Parish Nursing: Promoting Whole Person Health within Faith Communities* (New York: Sage Publication, 1999).

7. P. Ann Solari-Twadell, Anne Marie Djupe, and Mary Ann McDermott, eds., *Parish Nursing: The Developing Practice.* (Park Ridge, IL: National Parish Nurse Resource Center, 1990). A third text was P. Ann Solari-Twadell and Mary Ann McDermott, eds., *Parish Nursing: Development, Education and Administration.* (Elsevier Heatlh Sciences, 2006).

Chapter 25: Epilogue: Granger's Legacy

1. Interview of Ann Solari-Twadell by Jane Westberg, 1997.
2. For a brief history of the Association of Professional Chaplains as well as current activities see www.professionalchaplains.org
3. H. G. Koenig, E. G. Hooten, E. Lindsay-Calkins, and K. G. Meador. "Spirituality in Medical School Curricula: Findings from a National Survey," *The International Journal of Psychiatry in Medicine* 40, no. 4 (2010): 391–8.
4. Granger Westberg with Jill Westberg, *The Parish Nurse: How to Start a Parish Nurse Program in Your Church* (Park Ridge, Illinois: Parish Nurse Resource Center, 1987).
5. Lewis M. Andrews, "From Churches, A New Kind of Healing. Report from the Trenches," *The Wall Street Journal*, July 5, 1994.
6. Hilliard Jason and Andrew Douglas. "Are the Conditions Now Right for a 21st Century Medical School?" *The Lancet*, 385: 672–673, February 21, 2015.
7. Jill Westberg McNamara, *Health & Wellness* (Cleveland: The Pilgrim Press, 2006). Jill Westberg McNamara, *Stronger Together: Starting a Health Team in Your Congregation.* (Memphis: Church Health Center, 2013).

Bibliography

"Academy of Parish Clergy Founded," *The Christian Century*, 1969, 704.

American Nursing Association and Health Ministries Association, *Scope and Standards of Practice: Faith Community Nursing*, 2nd ed. (Silver Springs, MD: American Nurses Association, 2012).

Arden, G. Everett. *The School of the Prophets: The Background and History of Augustana Theological Seminary, 1860–1960*, Rock Island: IL: Augustana Theological Seminary, 1960.

Arden, G. Everett. *Augustana Heritage: A History of the Augustana Lutheran Church*. Rock Island, IL: Augustana Press, 1963.

Boisen, Anton *Exploration of the Inner Life: A Study of Mental Disorder and Religious Experience*. Philadelphia: University of Pennsylvania, 1971.

Byrd, Julian and Arne K. Jessen. "The College of Chaplains of the American Protestant Health Association." *Journal of Pastoral Care* 42, no. 3 (Fall 1988): 228–30.

Cabot, Richard and Russell Dicks. *The Art of Ministering to the Sick*, New York: Macmillan, 1936.

Clinebell, Howard J. *Community Mental Health—the Role of Church and Temple* (New York: Abingdon Press 1970). Chapter 28 Online: <www.religion-online.org/showchapter.asp?tit.le=798&C=1025>

Coates, Ta-Nehisi. "The Case for Reparations." *The Atlantic*, June 2014.

Cunningham, Robert M. *The Wholistic Health Centers: A New Direction in Health Care*. Battle Creek, MI: W. K. Kellogg Foundation, 1977.

Dicks, Russell L. "The Art of Ministering to the Sick." *Pastoral Psychology*, November 1952, 10.

Dicks, Russell L. "The Hospital Chaplain." *Pastoral Psychology*, April 1950, 50–54.

Geiser, Floramae. "Clinic in a Choir Room," *The Lutheran* (December, 1985): 15–16.

Grace, Helen K. "Nursing" In *Handbook of Health Professions Education*, edited by Christine H. McGuire, Richard Foley, Alan Gorr, Ronald W. Richards et al. San Francisco: Jossey-Bass Publishers, 1983.

Gurin G., J. Veroff and S. Feld, *Americans View Their Mental Health: A Nationwide Interview Survey*. NY: Basic Books, 1960.

Hiltner, Seward. "Man of the Month: Granger Westberg," *Pastoral Psychology*, August 1955, 6, 66.

Hiltner, Seward. *Pastoral Counseling*. Nashville, Tennessee: Abingdon Press, 1949.

Hiltner, Seward. *Religion and Health*. New York: Macmillan Company, 1943.

Hiltner, Seward. Review of *Minister and Doctor Meet*, *The Journal of Religion* (1961): 300.

Hofman, Hans, ed. *The Ministry and Mental Health*. New York: Association Press, 1960.

Holifield, E. Brooks. *A History of Pastoral Care in America: From Salvation to Self-Realization*. Nashville: Abingdon Press, 1983.

Holinger, Paul C., and Granger E. Westberg. "The Parish Pastor's Finest Hour—Revisited." *Journal of Religion and Health* 14, no. 4 (1975): 14–21.

Holst, Lawrence E. "The Parish Nurse," *Chronicle of Pastoral Care*. 7, Spring/Summer 1987, 13–17.

Joyce, Jon L. "Healing Body and Spirit." *The Lutheran*, March 3, 1971, 12–14.

Jason, Hilliard and Andrew Douglas. "Are the Conditions Now Right for a 21st Century Medical School?" *The Lancet* (February 21, 2015): 385: 672–673.

Kemper, Robert Graham. "Granger Westberg on Pastoral Care," *The Christian Ministry* 3, no. 4 (July, 1972): 15–17, 42–44.

Koenig H. G., E. G. Hooten, E. Lindsay-Calkins, K. G. Meador. "Spirituality in Medical School Curricula: Findings from a National Survey." *The International Journal of Psychiatry in Medicine* 40, no. 4 (2010): 391–8.

Lindemann, Erich. "Symptomatology and the Management of Acute Grief." *The American Journal of Psychiatry* 101 (September, 1944): 141–148.

"Man of the Month: Seward Hiltner." *Pastoral Psychology* 2, no. 13 (April 15, 1951): 1, 65.

McDermott, M. A., P. A. Solari-Twadell and R. Matheus. "Promoting Quality Education for the Parish Nurse and the Parish Nurse Coordinator" *Nursing and Health Care Perspective* 19, no. 1 (January/February 1998): 4–6.

McNamara, Jill Westberg. *Health & Wellness*. Cleveland: The Pilgrim Press, 2006.

McNamara, Jill Westberg, *Stronger Together: Starting a Health Team in Your Congregation*. Memphis, TN: Church Health Center, 2013.

Oates, Wayne. Review of *Minister and Doctor Meet*. *Pastoral Psychology*, June 1961, 55–56.

Peachey, Kirsten and Charles D. Phillips. "The College of Chaplains: The First 25 Years." *The Caregiver Journal* 12, no. 1 (1996): 6–17.

Peterson, William, ed., *Granger Westberg Verbatim: A Vision for Faith and Health*. St. Louis: International Parish Nurse Resource Center.

Rödlach, A. "Faith Community Nursing: An Emerging Ministry of Health and Healing Within the Church," *Verbum* 54, no. 2 (2013): 139–165.

Rogers, Carl. *Counseling and Psychotherapy*. Boston: Houghton Mifflin Company, 1942.

Rogers, Carl. "Through the Eyes of the Client," *Pastoral Psychology* 1, no. 2 (March 1950): 66.

Schultz, Charles M. *Good Grief, Charlie Brown*. Robinsdale, MN: Fawcett Publication, 1963.

Solari-Twadell, P. A. and M. A. McDermott. *Parish Nursing: Promoting Whole Person Health Within Faith Communities*. New York: Sage, 1999.

Starr, Paul. *The Social Transformation of American Medicine*. New York: Basic Books, Inc., 1982.

Stephenson, George M. *The Religious Aspects of Swedish Immigration*. Minneapolis: University of Minnesota Press, 1932.

Tengwald, V. J. "A Unique Church Mission," *The Lutheran Companion* (1941): 2–3.

Thornton, Edward E. *Professional Education for Ministry: A History of Clinical Pastoral Education*. Nashville: Abingdon Press, 1970.

Tubesing, Donald. *Whole Person Health Care An Idea in Evolution: History of the Wholistic Health Centers Project 1970-1976*. Hinsdale, IL: Wholistic Health Centers Inc., 1976.

Tubesing, Donald, Paul C. Holinger, Granger E. Westberg, and Edward Lichter, "The Wholistic Health Center Project: An Action-Research Model for Providing Preventive, Whole-Person Health Care at the Primary Level." *Medical Care* 15, no. 3 (1977): 217.

Tubesing, Don. *The Wholistic Health Centers: A New Direction in Health Care*, 1977.

Uehling, Carl T. "Ohio: A New Style Seminary," *The Lutheran*, June 18, 1969, 5–9.

Wendell , C. A. *The Larger Vision· A Study of the Evolution Theory in Its Relation to the Christian Faith*. Minneapolis, MN: self-published, 1925.

Westberg, Granger. "The Art of Worship." *The Lutheran Companion*, May 30, 1936, 684–685.

Westberg, Granger. "Marry Us, Reverend." *The Lutheran Companion*, July 31, 1941. Reprinted in *Religious Digest,* September, 1941, 50–52.

Westberg, Granger. "The Pulpit: The Growth of the Kingdom." *The Lutheran Companion*, January 29, 1942, 133–4.

Westberg, Granger. "Are Church Hospitals Different?" *The Augustana Quarterly* 12, no. 1 (January 1943): 53–63.

Westberg, Granger. "Pioneering in Church Hospitals." *The Lutheran Outlook,* May1943, 80–82.

Westberg, Granger. "Have You Ever Tried Counseling?" *The Lutheran Outlook*, September 1944. Reprinted in *Religious Digest*, November 1944, 71–74.

Westberg, Granger. "A Seminar in a Hospital." *The Lutheran Companion*, August 1, 1945, 8–9.

Westberg, Granger. "Will They Be Happy? A Guide to Marriage." *The Lutheran Companion*, February 2, 1949, 6–7.

Westberg, Granger. "Ministering to the Sick." *Central Conference American Rabbis Journal* 2 (1953): 28–33.

Westberg, Granger. "The Chaplain in the Modern Hospital." *The Bulletin of*

Maternal Welfare, March/April 1954, 11–13.

Westberg, Granger. "The Hospital Chaplain." Manuscript sent to Vergilius Ferm April 1954.

Westberg, Granger. "A Next Step in Ecumenicity." Sermon at Rockefeller Memorial Chapel February 27, 1955.

Westberg, Granger. "The Nurse Is the Chaplain's Ally." *The Modern Hospital* 84, no. 4 (April 1955): 82, 137

Westberg, Granger. "The Spiritual Needs of the Patient." *Parish Nurse Digest* 3 (September 1955): 16, 30.

Westberg, Granger. *Nurse, Pastor, and Patient: A Hospital Chaplain Talks to Nurses*. Rock Island, IL: Augustana Book Concern, 1955.

Westberg, Granger. "The Interrelationship of the Ministry and Medicine." *Pastoral Psychology*, April 1957, 9–13, 55.

Westberg, Granger. "Religious Aspects of Medical Teaching." *Journal of Medical Education* 32, no. 3 (March 1957): 204–209.

Westberg, Granger. "The "New" Field of Religion and Medicine." *Postgraduate Medicine* 23, no. 6 (1958): 668–71.

Westberg, Granger. "Advice to the Family on Being Given Diagnosis of Cancer." *Medical Clinics of North America* 42, no. 2 (March 1958): 563–568.

Westberg, Granger. "Are Ministers in a Rut?" *Augustana Seminary Review* 11, no. 2 (1959): 20–24.

Westberg, Granger. "The Role of the Clergyman in Mental Health." *Pastoral Psychology*, May 1960, 19–22.

Westberg, Granger. "The Need for Radical Changes in Theological Education: A Proposed 44-month Plan." In *The Ministry and Mental Health*, edited by Hans Hofman, 167–182. New York: Association Press, 1960.

Westberg, Granger. *Minister and Doctor Meet*. New York: Harper and Row, 1961.

Westberg, Granger. "Good Grief." *Trustee*, June 1962: 26–30

Westberg, Granger. *Good Grief*. Philadelphia: Fortress Press, 1962.

Westberg, Granger "Good Grief." *Christian Herald*, January 1964, 19–21.

Westberg, Granger. *Sjuksköterskan, Prästen och Patienten*. Stockholm: Diakonistyr, 1962.

Westberg, Granger. "Specific Jobs for Laymen." *The Lutheran*, July 29, 1964, 18–21.

Westberg, Granger. "A Medical Setting for Clergy Education." *Journal of Medical Education* 39 (October 1964): 953–58.

Westberg, Granger. "An American Academy of Parish Clergy: Why Not?" *Christian Century*, April 1965.

Westberg, Granger. "The Crucial First Three Minutes in the Sick Room." *Pastoral Psychology* (1965): 45–46.

Westberg, Granger, and Edgar Draper. *Community Psychiatry and the Clergyman*. Springfield, IL: Charles C. Thomas, 1966.

Westberg, Granger. "The Three Acts of Illness." *Christian Living*, February 1967, 8–10.

Westberg, Granger. "An Academy for Parish Clergy." *The Hamma Bulletin* 7, no. 3 (1969): 20–21.

Westberg, Granger. "The Risk of Openness." *The Hamma Bulletin.* 7, no. 1 (1969): 12–18.

Westberg, Granger. "Contextual Teaching of Pastoral Care in a Neighborhood Church Clinic." In *Explorations in Ministry: A Report on the Ministry in the 70's (Seventies) Project,* edited by Louis Douglass, 174–190. New York: IDOC-North America, 1971.

Westberg, Granger. "The Parish Pastor's Finest Hour." *Journal of Religion and Health,* April 1970, 171–84.

Westberg, Granger. "Parish Clergymen and Mental Health: The Kokomo and La Grange Projects." In *The Role of Church and Temple*, edited by Howard J Clinebell. New York: Abingdon Press, 1970. Available online <http://www.religion-online,org/showchapter.asp?title=798&C=1025>

Westberg, Granger. *How to Start a Church-Based Clinic.* Charles F. Kettering Foundation, 1975.

Westberg, Granger. "Can the Clergy Help Overworked Physicians? Experiences with an Experimental Church Clinic." *Postgraduate Medicine* 53, no. 7 (June 1973): 165–67.

Westberg, Granger. "From Hospital Chaplaincy to Wholistic Health Center." *The Journal of Pastoral Care* 33, no. 2 (1979): 76–82.

Westberg, Granger. "The Growing Role of Clergy in Wholistic Medicine." AMHC Forum 32, no. 2 (1979): 38–47.

Westberg, Granger. *Theological Roots of Wholistic Health Care. A Response to the Religious Questions that Have Been Raised.* Hinsdale, IL: Wholistic Health Center, Inc., 1979.

Westberg, Granger. "The Church as a Health Place." *Dialog* 27, no. 3 (1982): 189–191.

Westberg. Granger. "Churches Are Joining the Health Care Team." *Urban Health,* October, 1984, 34–36.

Westberg, Granger. "Nurses as 'Ministers of Health,'" August 1985.

Westberg, Granger. "The Role of Congregations in Preventive Medicine," *Journal of Religion and Health* 25, no. 3 (September 1986): 193–197.

Westberg, Granger. "Why Me, Lord." *The Lutheran*, September 1986, 5–62.

Westberg, Granger. "Why Me, Lord." *The Disciple* 13, no. 9 (May 21, 1986): 20–22

Westberg, Granger with Jill Westberg. *The Parish Nurse: How to Start a Parish Nurse Program in Your Church.* Park Ridge, IL: Parish Nurse Resource Center, 1987.

Westberg, Granger. "Preventive Medicine." *Entrée*, April 1987, 11–13.

Westberg, Granger. "The Church as "Health Place,'" *Dialog: A Journal of Theology* 27, no. 3 (Winter 1988): 189–195.

Westberg, Granger. "Parishes, Nurses and Health Care." *Lutheran Partners,* November/December, 1988, 26–29.

Westberg, Granger. "Parish Nursing's Pioneer." *Journal of Christian Nursing* (Winter 1989): 26–29.

Westberg, Granger. "What a Congregation Looks Like that Takes Wholistic Health Seriously." In *Health Care and Its Costs: A Challenge for the Church,* edited by Walter E. Wiest. Lantham, New York, and London: University Press of America, 1988.

Westberg, Granger. "A New Vision of the Chaplain of Tomorrow from a Personal Friend of Russell Dicks." Russell L. Dicks Memorial Lecture, 1990.

Westberg, Granger with Jill Westberg McNamara, *The Parish Nurse: Providing a Minister of Health for Your Congregation.* Minneapolis: Augsburg, 1990.

Westberg, Granger. "A Personal Historical Perspective of Whole Person Health Care and the Congregation." In *Parish Nursing: Promoting Whole Person Health within Faith Communities,* edited by Patrician Ann Solari-Twadell and Mary Ann McDermott, 35–41. Thousand Oaks, CA: Sage Publication, 1999.

Westberg, Jill. "Hope." In *Theological Roots of Wholistic Health Care: A Response to the Religious Questions that Have Been Raised,* edited by Granger Westberg, 73–92. Hinsdale, IL: Wholistic Health Center, Inc., 1979.

The papers of Granger Westberg are archived at Loyolta University in Chicago, Illinois. www.luc.edu/media/lucedu/archives/pdfs/westberg2.pdf

Index

MORE BOOKS FROM CHURCH HEALTH

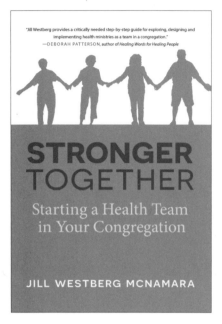

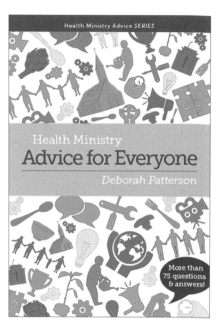

Stronger Together: Starting a Health Team in Your Congregation
By Jill Westberg McNamara

Health Ministry Advice for Everyone
By Deborah Patterson

It takes time and determination to develop a health ministry team, but a map through the process can make the route clearer. With a blend of organizational principles, practical tips, inspirational stories, and proven real-life program models in churches, *Stronger Together: Starting a Health Team in Your Congregation* is a valuable guide that your health team—whether just starting out or seeking new energy—will refer to again and again.

In *Health Ministry Advice for Everyone*, Deborah Patterson answers some of the most pressing or perplexing questions on health and wellness in congregations. Are you hitting a roadblock with a program in your church? Are you wondering where to start with health ministry? Do you feel like you need a new idea on a specific topic? This book provides in-depth advice from healthier coffee hours to walking programs to caregiver support.

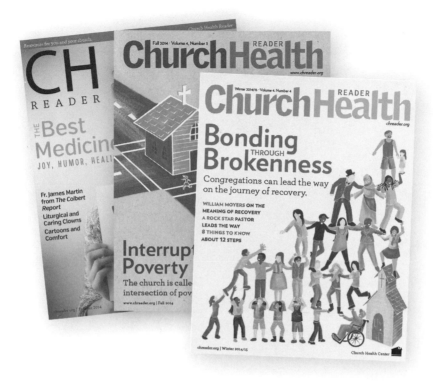